DRUGS HANDBOOK

1999

DRUGS HANDBOOK

1999

Glyn Volans Heather Wiseman

Twenty-first revised edition published 1998 by
MACMILLAN REFERENCE LTD, 1998
25 Eccleston Place, London, SW1W 9NF
and Basingstoke

Companies and representatives throughout the world.

http://www.macmillan-reference.co.uk

Distributed by
Macmillan Direct,
Brunel Road, Houndmills,
Basingstoke,
Hampshire, RG21 2XS, England

ISBN 0-333-69444-9

A catalogue record for this book is available from the British Library.

Typeset by EXPO Holdings, Malaysia

Printed and bound in the UK by
Antony Rowe Ltd, Chippenham, Wiltshire

DEDICATION

To the memory of our colleague, Professor Paul Turner, in recognition of his role in establishing and maintaining this book over a period of 18 years, and in appreciation of his experience and teaching that formed the basis for this work.

October 1998
GLYN N. VOLANS
HEATHER M. WISEMAN

CONTENTS

PREFACE

This revised edition contains new products introduced during the last year and has been fully revised to take account of withdrawals and revisions. The substances in the Approved Name Section are listed under their British Approved Names, but this year we have included Recommended International Non-proprietary Names (rINN) with cross-references to existing entries. The rINNs are being introduced to standardize drug nomenclature throughout the world, thereby improving communications about medicinal substances. They will eventually replace British Approved Names as a requirement of the European Directive 92/27/EEC. Readers have told us that they sometimes appreciate information on drugs which are no longer included in prescribed medication in the United Kingdom. For this reason we have retained some entries on drugs which are obsolete but still of therapeutic, toxicological or pharmacological interest. Readers have also expressed appreciation of the section of definitions of drug group names and medical terms, and we have therefore extended them further in this edition.

We have also been asked to give information on drugs that are misused or abused. We have done this by identifying them with the abbreviation (m) and have provided an Appendix of common slang names for misused drugs. We would like to thank the National Criminal Intelligence Service for providing some of these names.

We have considered taking account of the so-called limited list but think that it cannot be accommodated directly in this text in view of the number and frequency of the revisions to the list. For further information on this list the reader is referred to the relevant section in the Introduction.

October 1998
GLYN N. VOLANS
HEATHER M. WISEMAN

INTRODUCTION

Patient care has now extended far beyond the patient–doctor relationship and involves several different highly trained health care professions including, amongst others, nurses, midwives, occupational therapists, physiotherapists, radiographers, electro-encephalographers, dieticians, social workers, psychologists and medical secretaries. Although prescribing of medicines is the responsibility of a doctor, the drugs which medicines contain may influence patients in many ways, and it is important that others involved in a patient's health care should have ready access to information on the various medicines which he or she may receive, either by prescription or by over-the-counter purchase. The primary purpose of this book is to provide such information for these and other groups within the health professions. It is not a textbook of clinical pharmacology or medical treatment nor is it intended to be: rather it is meant to be a short guide to the mechanism of action, therapeutic indications and chief unwanted effects of most medicines available in the United Kingdom.

Drugs and Medicines

A doctor usually prescribes a *drug*, but the patient receives a *medicine*. The medicine is the whole formulation in which the drug, that is the active substance, is combined with other ingredients to form a convenient form of administration, such as a tablet, capsule, suppository, inhalation, ointment or injection. We have not included all constituents of the medicines listed in this book, but have mentioned only those substances which we believe may contribute to the therapeutic or adverse effects of the medicine involved. It must be stressed that the mention of a medicine in this book, and statements about its indications, do not imply that it is necessarily an effective treatment, or that the authors believe it to be such, in fact we believe that for large numbers of drugs there is no good evidence of their effectiveness.

Names of Drugs

Most drugs have at least three names. The first is the full chemical name, which is too long and complicated to use regularly. More convenient is the shorter *generic* or *approved* name, which may become accepted internationally. Finally, there is the *brand* or *trade* name, given by the pharmaceutical manufacturer for its own particular brand or formulation. For example, 4-amino-5-chloro-*N*-(2-diethylaminoethyl)-2-methoxybenzamide hydrochloride is the chemical name for metoclopramide hydrochloride, the approved name of the drug marketed at present by at least two drug firms under the brand names Maxolon and Primperan. We have distinguished between approved and brand names by compiling two separate alphabetical lists. The main body of the book is devoted to approved names, with a brand name index at the end, and to save space and avoid duplication of information almost all the brand names have been cross-referenced to the appropriate approved names. Also in the interests of saving space, where a number of drugs have essentially similar effects we have cross-referenced approved names to those which we consider to be the most typical and most frequently prescribed. Thus all cross-references refer to the list of approved names, and are shown in small capitals, for example, AMETHOCAINE.

Drugs in Pregnancy

Several drugs are known to be hazardous to the developing foetus and for most drugs there is no definite information on their safety in pregnancy. We have avoided constant repetition of this but would stress that in pregnancy all drugs should be used with caution and only when essential.

Drug Combinations

Many of the preparations listed in this book are combinations of drugs rather than individual ones. The majority are rather crude attempts at what might be called 'blunderbuss treatment' of a variety of signs and symptoms, but some have been developed on scientific grounds to exploit the interaction of two or more drugs working together. Others, by combining drugs that are commonly used together, offer, if correctly used, a means of simplifying treatment for patients on long-term multiple drugs and thus improve compliance, for example, combination drugs for hypertension. Several approved names have now been coined for such combinations. These are identified by the prefix 'co-', and usually include syllables from the approved names of the ingredient drugs. For example, co-trimoxazole is a combination of trimethoprim and sulphamethoxazole.

Limited List

In 1985 the government issued a 'black list' of drugs and preparations that cannot be prescribed or dispensed under the NHS but only on private prescriptions, the patient having to pay for them in full. These restrictions on prescribing and dispensing at the public expense are at present limited to the following therapeutic groups:

- Antacids
- Laxatives
- Analgesics used for mild or moderate pain
- Cough and cold remedies, which include cough suppressants, expectorants, mucolytics, inhalations, and nasal decongestants
- Tonics
- Vitamins
- Benzodiazepine tranquillizers, sedatives and hypnotics

An advisory committee has been set up to advise the Department of Health on changes that should be made in the list. Doctors and pharmacists are able to recognize which drugs and medicines cannot be prescribed under the NHS by a symbol published against their names in the *British National Formulary*.

Technical Terms, Further Information

This book has not been written for the general public, and it assumes a basic knowledge and understanding of human biology and disease. Many readers may, nevertheless, wish to refer to larger books for more complete and detailed information, and we would recommend:

1. For information on drugs

Laurence, D. R., Bennett, P. N. and Brown M. J. *Clinical Pharmacology.* 8th Edition. 1997. Churchill-Livingstone, London.
Reynolds, J. E. F. (Ed.) Martindale: *The Extra Pharmacopoeia.* 31st Edition, 1997. The Royal Pharmaceutical Society, London.
Hardman, J. G., Gilman, A. G., and Limbird, L. E. *Goodman & Gilman's The Pharmacological Basis of Therapeutics*. 9th Edition, 1996. McGraw-Hill, New York.
Reid, J. L., Rubin, P. C. and Whiting, B. *Lecture Notes on Clinical Pharmacology*. 5th Edition, 1996. Blackwell Science.
Ritter, J. M., Lewis, L. D., and Mant, T. G. K. *A Textbook of Clinical Pharmacology.* 3rd Edition, 1995. Edward Arnold, London.
Trounce J., *Clinical Pharmacology for Nurses*. 15th Edition, 1997. Churchill Livingstone, London.

2. For information on diseases and their management

Rees, P. J. and Williams, D. G. *Principles of Clinical Medicine*. 1995. Edward Arnold, London.
Kumar, P. J. and Clark, M. L. (Eds.) *Clinical Medicine.* 3rd Edition. 1994. Baillière Tindall, London.

3. For information on treatment of poisoning

Bates, N., Edwards, J. N., Roper, J., Volans, G. N. (Eds.) *Paediatric Toxicology*. 1997. Macmillan, London.
Ellenhorn, M. J. *Ellenhorn's Medical Toxicology*. 2nd Edition, 1997. Williams & Wilkins, Baltimore.

October 1998
GLYN N. VOLANS
HEATHER M. WISEMAN

ABBREVIATIONS

The following abbreviations have been used throughout the book:

(b) indicates a borderline substance, that is a substance which may only be prescribed as a drug under certain conditions.

(c) indicates a drug whose prescription is controlled under the Misuse of Drugs Act.

(d) discontinued by the manufacturers during the year prior to publication. As supplies will still be available from pharmacies until stocks run out, these products have not yet been deleted from our lists.

(m) indicates a drug that is misused or abused, although not controlled by the Misuse of Drugs Act.

CNS Central nervous system.

rINN Recommended International Non-proprietary Name

DEFINITIONS OF DRUG GROUP NAMES AND MEDICAL TERMS

abortifacient. Used to produce abortion.

adjuvant. Something added to a drug which aids or modifies the main ingredient.

adrenergic. Has similar actions to adrenaline.

adrenoceptor. Receptor for ADRENALINE, NORADRENALINE, which mediates sympathetic activity in the body.

adsorbent. Material which binds drugs and other chemicals and prevents or reduces their absorption.

agonist. Has an observable effect within the body, resulting from a direct action upon a specific receptor.

alpha-adrenoceptor. Subgroup of adrenoceptors that mediates some of the effects of sympathetic stimulation including vasoconstriction, increase in blood pressure and mydriasis.

amino acids. Simple molecules from which peptides, polypeptides and proteins are formed.

aminoglycoside. Drug with a chemical structure related to STREPTOMYCIN.

anabolic. Stimulates cell metabolism causing increased tissue growth.

analgesic. Relieves pain.

anorectic. Appetite suppressant used in obesity.

antacid. Neutralizes acid produced by the stomach.

antagonist. Opposes the action or blocks the effect of another drug.

antiandrogen. Acts to block the effects of the male sex hormones (androgens).

antiarrhythmic. Suppresses arrhythmias.

anticholinergic. Blocks the action of ACETYLCHOLINE or cholinergic (acetylcholine-like) drugs.

anticholinesterase. Blocks the action of cholinesterase – a naturally occurring enzyme which breaks down ACETYLCHOLINE bringing its action to an end. The effect of the anticholinesterase is therefore to prolong and intensify the action of acetylcholine.

anticoagulant. Prevents blood from clotting.

anticonvulsant. Stops or prevents epileptic seizures.

antidysrhythmic. *See* antiarrhythmic.

antiemetic. Prevents nausea and vomiting.

antihistamine. Blocks the action of histamine.

antihypertensive. Lowers blood pressure.

antipruritic. Relieves pruritus.

antipyretic. Lowers body temperature in febrile conditions.

antiserotonin. Blocks the action of serotonin.

antispasmodic. Relieves spasm of muscles, for example, in the gastro-intestinal tract (gastro-intestinal colic).

antitussive. Suppresses cough.

anxiolytic. Reduces anxiety.

arrhythmia. Disorder of rhythm, generally of the heart.

arthralgia. Pain in the joints.

asthenia. General feeling of physical weakness.

astringent. Precipitates protein to form a protective layer over damaged skin or mucous membranes.

bactericidal. Kills bacteria.

bacteriostatic. Inhibits growth of bacteria but does not kill them.

benzodiazepines. A group of chemically related hypnotics, sedatives, anxiolytics and anticonvulsants including DIAZEPAM.

beta-adrenoceptor. Subgroup of adrenoceptors that mediates some of the effects of sympathetic stimulation including increase in heart rate and force, and bronchodilation.

beta-lactam. An antibiotic with a chemical structure which includes a beta-lactam ring. CEPHALOSPORINS, PENICILLINS, and CEFOXITIN are beta-lactam antibiotics.

beta-lactamase. Enzyme produced by some bacteria, capable of breaking down the beta-lactam ring of the beta-lactam antibiotics. Leads to bacterial resistance to the antibiotic. Some beta-lactam antibiotics are beta-lactamase resistant, e.g. CLOXACILLIN.

bioavailability. Extent to which and rate at which the active substance in a drug is taken up by the body in a form that is physiologically active.

bradycardia. Slow heart rate.

bronchodilator. Increases the diameter of the airways in the respiratory system and thus reduces the physical resistance to breathing.

buffer. Solution that opposes changes in acidity or alkalinity.

cardioselective. Acts on the heart without the other effects usually found in drugs of a particular group, for example beta-adrenoceptor blocking drugs. In practice, the cardioselectivity is usually relative and the other effects can be traced, although in a less pronounced form.

carminative. Facilitates the eructation of gas from the stomach.

cathartic. Relieves constipation.

chelating agents. Bind heavy metals to increase their excretion.

chemotherapy. Treatment using drugs rather than other measures such as surgery, radiation or vaccines.

cholinergic. Has actions similar to ACETYLCHOLINE

corticosteroids. Hormones (natural or synthetic) with actions on metabolism and against tissue inflammation. The natural hormones are produced by the adrenal gland.

cutaneous. Relating to the skin.

cycloplegic. Paralyses muscle of the eye controlling accommodation. Leads to blurred vision.

cytotoxic. Has toxic effects upon living cells which reduce growth or cause destruction of the cells.

decongestant. Reduces congestion (i.e. swelling) of the nasal mucosa.

delirium. A state of impaired consciousness, and mental confusion.

demulcent. Supposed to coat and smooth mucous membranes of the gastro-intestinal tract (e.g., milk, raw egg white).

dermatitis. General term to describe inflammation of the skin, which may be due to many causes.

diuretic. Increases urine output.

dyspepsia. Indigestion.

elixir. Clear, flavoured liquid preparation of drug frequently containing alcohol and sweetening and colouring agents.

embolus. Mobile blood clot which travels through the bloodstream until it wedges in a blood vessel and blocks the blood supply to the part of the body supplied by that vessel.

embrocation. A liquid formulation for external application on, or rubbing into, a diseased or painful joint or muscle.

emetic. Induces vomiting.

emollient. Topical softening application.

encephalitis. Inflammation of brain tissue.

encephalopathy. Comprehensive term to describe general abnormality of brain tissue function. May be due to many causes.

endogenous. Produced or found within the body.

endometriosis. 'Islands' of uterine lining cells scattered throughout the other abdominal organs. Symptoms include abdominal pain and heavy menstruation.

enema. Drug formulation for rectal administration.

enteric coating. Surface coating of capsules or tablets designed to resist gastric acid acting on it, so that the drug is not released until reaching the small intestine.

enzyme. A reactive protein which mediates a chemical reaction without itself being altered.

essential oil. Volatile oil derived by distillation from part of a plant.

exogenous. Derived from outside the body.

expectorant. Aids removal of sputum from the lungs and respiratory passages.

febrifuge. A preparation that lowers raised body temperature (fever).

fibrinolytic. Dissolves or otherwise destroys the fibrin which is formed when blood clots.

GABA (Gaba amino butyric acid). Inhibitory neurotransmitter found in the brain. Reduced activity is associated with epilepsy, hence drugs which enhance GABA effects may be used as anticonvulsants.

G6PD. Glucose 6-phosphate dehydrogenase: an enzyme involved in carbohydrate metabolism. Some patients exhibit an inherited deficiency of this enzyme and are thus more susceptible to certain diseases and adverse drug effects.

galactorrhoea. Inappropriate production of breast milk in either sex, not associated with a recent pregnancy.

gel. Jelly-like formulation of medicinal ingredients.

gynaecomastia. Abnormal enlargement of the breasts in men.

haematinic. Involved in the normal development of red blood cells.

haemolysis. Increased breakdown of red blood cells.

haemorrhoids. Piles.

haemostatic. Reduces or stops blood loss.

herbicide. Kills plants.

hirsutism. Increased and extensive hair growth.

hormone. Naturally occurring substance which is secreted by a gland into the blood stream, whence it is carried to the part of the body on which it acts. Insulin, for example, is secreted by the pancreas and acts at sites all over the body.

HRT. Hormone replacement therapy for relief of menopausal/post-menopausal symptoms. Uses small doses of the hormones used for contraception.

hyperaldosteronism. Excessive secretion of the salt-retaining hormone ALDOSTERONE.

hypercalcaemia. Raised serum calcium above normal levels.

hyperglycaemia. Raised blood glucose above normal levels.

hyperkalaemia. Raised serum potassium above normal levels.

hyperlipidaemia. High concentrations of lipids (fats) in the blood, measured as cholesterol and triglycerides. May be inherited, acquired (dietary), or a mixture of both. Untreated hyperlipidaemias are associated with atherosclerotic disease, leading to heart attacks, strokes and poor blood supply to the legs and other parts of the body. Treatment consists of reduction of dietary fat intake, plus lipid lowering drugs, if necessary.

hypernatraemia. Raised serum sodium above normal levels.

hyperthyroidism. Abnormal increase in thyroid function.

hypnotic. Facilitates sleep.

hypocalcaemia. Reduced serum calcium below normal levels.

hypoglycaemia. Reduced blood glucose below normal levels.

hypokalaemia. Reduced serum potassium below normal levels.

hyponatraemia. Reduced serum sodium below normal levels.

hypotensive. Lowers blood pressure.

hypothyroidism. Abnormal decrease in thyroid function.

immunosuppressant. Tends to suppress the immune response. This effect may be used to suppress some cancers or rejection of transplanted organs, but it makes the body more susceptible to infections.

infusion. Administration of a drug by continuous intravenous drip/injection.

insecticide. Kills insects.

insomnia. Lack of, or inability to, sleep.

isomer. One of two or more molecules having the same number and kind of atoms but differing in the arrangement or configuration of the atoms. Optical isomers are compounds whose structures are mirror images of each other. Isomers may differ in the order in which atoms are joined together, or in the position of atoms or groups of atoms in the molecule.

When a drug exists in more than one isomer, one isomer may have all or most of the pharmacological activity. Recent trends in drug development include the introduction of specific isomers rather than the normal racemic mixtures.

keratolytic. Removes dry scaly skin.

laxative. Relieves constipation.

linctus. Viscous liquid preparation of drug containing sugar or alternative sweetening agent.

liniment. A liquid formulation for external application on, or rubbing into, a diseased or painful joint or muscle.

lotion. Wet dressing used to cleanse and cool inflamed skin lesions.

lozenge. Tablet, originally diamond shape, of flavoured medication to be dissolved in the mouth.

melaena. Black stools due to passage of altered blood from haemorrhage.

meningitis. Inflammation of the meninges, the covering of the brain.

miotic. Constricts the pupil of the eye.

mucolytic. Liquifies mucus within the respiratory system.

myalgia. Pain in muscles.

mydriatic. Dilates the pupil of the eye.

narcotic analgesic. Pain-relieving drug of the opium group. Liable to have addictive properties.

nephritis. Inflammation of kidney tissue.

nephrotoxic. Causes damage to the kidneys.

neuropathy. Comprehensive term to describe general abnormality of function of a peripheral nerve, which may be due to many causes.

neurotransmitter. Biochemical substance which acts in the transmission of nerve impulses.

neutrophil. One of the families of white blood cells which is involved in combating bacterial infection.

oedema. Swelling and congestion of tissues due to accumulation of fluid derived from the blood plasma.

ototoxic. Causes damage to nerves involved in hearing.

parasympatholytic. Antagonises the action of ACETYLCHOLINE. *See* ANTICHOLINERGIC.

parasympathomimetic. Has actions similar to the parasympathetic chemical transmitter in the nervous system ACETYLCHOLINE.

parenteral. Administered by a route other than via the gastro-intestinal tract. Usually refers to intradermal, subcutaneous, intramuscular or intravenous injection.

pastille. A sweetened medicinal formulation with a round flat shape, to be dissolved in the mouth.

peptide. A chain of amino acids.

pessary. Solid-dose drug formulation similar to suppository but placed in the vagina. Usually used for local actions in the vagina but systemic absorption of the drug may occur.

pesticide. Kills pests. This term includes a wide range of compounds (e.g., rodenticides which kill rats and small mammals, insecticides, herbicides).

Only a few of these chemicals also have applications as drugs.

pharmaceutical aid. An ingredient used to produce a convenient formulation of a drug for administration by a particular route.

pharmacodynamics. Study of the actions of drugs in living systems.

pharmacokinetics. Study of the fate of drugs in the body. Includes absorption, distribution, metabolism and excretion.

phenothiazine. Drug with a chemical structure similar to CHLORPROMAZINE.

phosphodiesterase. Enzyme, the inhibition of which leads to effects similar to beta-adrenoceptor stimulation.

photophobia. Intolerance to light.

placebo. Inactive substance or preparation used in controlled studies to evaluate the effectiveness of a medicinal substance. In some instances, a placebo may be prescribed to satisfy the patient's desire for medicine. In other instances, a supposedly 'active' drug may be prescribed but the benefits seen relate not to this action but to the 'placebo' effect.

plasma. The cell-free fluid component of the blood.

plasmin. An enzyme which acts on fibrin in small clots in blood vessels with the result that the clot dissolves and disintegrates.

pneumonitis. Inflammation of the tissues of the lung.

polypeptide. A complex molecule made up of peptides.

polysaccharide. A complex sugar molecule.

prodrug. A chemical that is converted into an active drug within the body.

prokinetic. Facilitates movement throughout the gastro-intestinal tract by increasing contractions of the gut wall.

prophylactic. Tends to prevent a condition rather than treat it when established.

prostaglandins. A group of very active substances found throughout the body with a large number of actions including effects on the uterus, airways, and blood vessels.

protein. A complex molecule made up of polypeptides.

pruritis. Persistent itching.

psychosis. Major disturbance in mental function, with abnormalities in thought processes often accompanied by hallucinations.

purgative. Facilitates evacuation of the bowels.

purine nucleoside. A chemical related to the basic protein structure of which chromosomes are constructed.

receptor. Site on cell surfaces which reacts to drugs or endogenous substance to produce the observed effect.

retinitis. Inflammation of the retina, the layer of nerve cells at the back of the eye which senses light impulses and mediates vision.

retrobulbar neuritis. Inflammation of the optic nerve between the brain and eye.

rhinitis. Inflammation of the nasal passages.

rub. A formulation for topical application.

rubefacient. Causes reddening of the skin.

sclerosing agent. Produces an inflammatory reaction and fibrosis, leading to closure of blood vessels.

sedative. Reduces arousal.

sinus rhythm. The normal regular heart rhythm.

suppository. Solid-dose, elongated, cone-shaped drug formulation for insertion into the rectum for local treatment (e.g., for haemorrhoids) or for drug absorption (e.g., antiemetic). Has a fatty base which melts at body temperature.

sustained-release formulation. Product specifically designed to release the active drug more slowly and over a prolonged period. Used to increase the interval between doses and to prevent toxicity from high drug concentrations achieved in the body when there is rapid absorption.

sympathomimetic. Has actions similar to the chemical transmitters of sympathetic nervous system (ADRENALINE and NORADRENALINE).

tachycardia. Rapid heart rate.

tachyphylaxis. Occurs when repeated doses of the drug produce progressively smaller effects (or else progressively bigger doses are required).

tardive dyskinesia. A neurological syndrome associated with long-term use of dopamine receptor blocking antipsychotic drugs such as phenothiazines, and characterized by involuntary movements.

teratogenic. May produce congenital malformation if given during the first three months of pregnancy.

thiazide. Drug with a chemical structure similar to CHLOROTHIAZIDE.

thrombolytic. Breaks down clots in the vascular system.

thrombophlebitis. Formation of clot in an inflamed vein.

thrombus. Blood clot.

tolerance. Has the same meaning as tachyphylaxis (see above).

topical. Applied externally at the site where the drug action is needed (e.g., for treatment of skin rashes or eye infections).

toxoid. A preparation of a bacterial toxin that has its toxic properties removed but has retained its ability to stimulate the body's immunity to it by the production of antibodies.

tranquillizer. Drug with sedative actions on the brain which is used in the treatment and management of certain psychiatric disorders, for example, schizophrenia, mania.

vaccine. Preparation of live attenuated or dead micro-organisms used to induce immunity.

vasoconstrictor. Causes constriction of blood vessels.

vasodilator. Causes dilatation of blood vessels.

vitamin. Chemical essential in small amounts for maintenance of normal growth and health. Must be obtained from external sources, usually dietary. Inadequate intake leads to deficiency diseases.

PART I

Approved Names

A

Abciximab. Monoclonal antibody which binds to receptors on the walls of blood vessels and thus blocks the formation of a blood platelet clot. Used in non-invasive heart surgery (angioplasty) to reduce the risk of blood clots forming after the operation and to reduce risk of myocardial infarct in patients with unstable angina. May cause bleeding complications and should not be used in any patient with a previous history of such problems.

Acamprosate. Analogue of the neurotransmitter GABA. Used to aid abstinence in chronic alcoholism, where it acts on GABA receptors to reduce craving for alcohol. May cause gastro-intestinal disturbance, skin reactions and fluctuations in libido.

Acarbose. Saccharide that inhibits the digestive enzyme alpha-glucosidase which breaks dietary carbohydrate down to monosaccharides. This leads to a reduction in blood glucose level. Indicated in patients with non-insulin dependent diabetes who are inadequately controlled by diet alone, or in combination with other oral drug treatment. Adverse effects include flatulence and diarrhoea.

Acebutolol. Beta-adrenoceptor blocking drug, with limited cardioselectivity. Uses, side effects, etc. as for PROPRANOLOL.

Aceclofenac. Non-steroidal anti-inflammatory analgesic with actions, uses and adverse effects similar to DICLOFENAC.

Acemetacin. Non-steroid anti-inflammatory/analgesic used in treatment of rheumatoid arthritis, osteoarthritis and post-operative pain and inflammation. Adverse effects include gastro-intestinal symptoms, headache, dizziness, oedema, chest pain, pruritus, blood dyscrasias, tinnitus, and blurred vision.

Acenocoumarol. rINN for NICOUMALONE.

Acetaminophen. USA: *see* PARACETAMOL.

Acetazolamide. Weak diuretic. Also used in glaucoma to reduce intraocular pressure, and as an anticonvulsant. Acts by inhibiting carbonic anhydrase and so reduces hydrogen ions available for exchange with sodium ions. May cause drowsiness, mental confusion, and paraesthesia.

Acetomenaphthone. *See* VITAMIN K.

Acetylcholine. Neurotransmitter, particularly in parasympathetic system. Peripheral effects include miosis, paralysis of accommodation, increased glandular secretions, contraction of smooth muscle in gastro-intestinal, respiratory and urogenital systems, slowing of heart, and vasodilatation. These effects blocked by ATROPINE SULPHATE. Not used clinically.

Acetylcysteine. Mucolytic. Administered by mouth or by inhalation from a nebulizer. Liquefies mucus and aids expectoration in diseases where mucus is troublesome (e.g., chronic bronchitis). May cause bronchospasm, haemoptysis. nausea, and vomiting. Used also in lubricant eye drops and intravenously in the treatment of PARACETAMOL overdosage where it prevents liver damage by restoring or acting as a substitute for depleted liver glutathione stores. In this use may also cause rash, nausea, vomiting, and transient bronchospasm.

Acetylsalicylic acid (Aspirin). Anti-inflammatory, antipyretic analgesic. Inhibits prostaglandin synthesis, reduces stickiness of blood platelets. Used to reduce risk of stroke and of heart attacks. May cause gastric erosion and haemorrhage, hypersensitivity reactions. Tinnitus and hyperventilation leading to respiratory and cardiovascular failure in overdose. Interacts with oral anticoagulants and sulphonylureas. Forced alkaline diuresis may be used to speed elimination in overdosage.

Aciclovir. Antiviral agent used orally, topically and intravenously to treat herpes simplex and varicella-zoster infections. Should not be used when patient is dehydrated as may cause rise in blood urea and creatinine.

Acipimox. Reduces raised blood lipids by inhibiting the release of fatty acids from fat tissue. Related chemically to NICOTINIC ACID. Adverse reactions include flushing and headache.

Acitretin. The major metabolite of ETRETINATE with similar actions, adverse reactions and contraindications. Patients are advised to avoid alcohol because of increased risk of effects on the foetus.

Aclarubicin. Cytotoxic antibiotic used in treatment of leukaemia. Adverse effects include bone marrow suppression, phlebitis and cardiotoxicity. Related to DAUNORUBICIN but may act by a different mechanism and appears to cause less cardiotoxicity.

Acrivastine. Antihistamine for treatment of allergies and hay fever. It is fast-acting and has a short duration of action. It seldom causes drowsiness.

Acrosoxacin. Antibiotic used only in treatment of gonorrhoea where the patient is allergic to PENICILLIN or organism is resistant to penicillins and other antibiotics. Needs only single dose. May cause dizziness, drowsiness, headache, and gastrointestinal disturbances.

Actinomycin D. Cytotoxic antibiotic used in neoplastic disease. Adverse effects include bone marrow depression.

Activated charcoal. Charcoal is a strong adsorbent. 'Activated' indicates simply that the charcoal meets certain standards in adsorbence tests. Used by mouth in cases of acute poisoning to reduce absorption of drugs or other toxins. May cause nausea and vomiting. Would adsorb oral emetics or antidotes and therefore should not be used if these are given. Subsequent black stools should not be mistaken for melaena.

Activated dimethicone. Liquid silicone polymer (dimethicone) plus finely divided silicon dioxide used as an antifoaming agent to relieve gas bubbles from gastrointestinal tract (e.g., in flatulence or dyspepsia).

Adapalene. Vitamin A analogue with actions and adverse effects similar to TRETINOIN. Used in topical treatment of severe acne.

Adenosine. Endogenous purine nucleoside which acts on specific receptors in heart muscle and coronary arteries to reduce heart rate. Given by intravenous injection to assist in diagnosis of certain fast heart rhythms and to convert some fast rhythms back to normal 'sinus' rhythm. May cause facial flushing, sweating, burning sensations, chest pain, palpitations, heart block, shortness of breath, headaches and blurred vision.

Adenosine monophosphoric acid (AMP). Source of high-energy phosphate bonds for tissue metabolism. Suggested for use in cardiovascular disease and rheumatism but efficacy unproven.

Adenosine triphosphoric acid (ATP). Source of high-energy phosphate bonds for tissue metabolism. Suggested for use in cardiovascular disease and rheumatism but efficacy unproven.

Adrenaline. Sympathomimetic amine, alpha- and beta-adrenoceptor agonist. Produces vasoconstriction with rise in blood pressure, cardioacceleration and bronchodilation. Used in acute allergic reactions, as peripheral vasoconstrictor, in narrow-angle glaucoma and in cardiac arrest. Toxicity includes hypertension, pulmonary oedema, and cardiac arrhythmias.

Agar. Purgative. Increases faecal bulk by same mechanism as METHYLCELLULOSE but less effective.

Alclofenac. Anti-inflammatory analgesic with actions similar to IBUPROFEN.

Alclometasone. Topical corticosteroid for treatment of eczema and other non-infective inflammatory conditions. Actions and adverse effects similar to HYDROCORTISONE.

Aldesleukin. Growth factor produced by recombinant techniques, involved in regulation of normal growth and differentiation of cells involved in immune mechanisms. Used in treatment of renal cancer which has spread throughout the body. Given intravenously, it produces many unwanted effects including fever, rigor, weight gain and hypotension.

Aldosterone. Naturally occurring adrenal (mineralocorticoid) steroid hormone. Acts mainly on salt and water metabolism by increasing salt retention in the kidney; has no useful anti-inflammatory activity. Used only in replacement therapy for adrenal insufficiency.

Alendronate. A biphosphonate with actions on remodelling of bone similar to ETIDRONATE. Use to treat osteoporosis in post-menopausal women. May cause abdominal pain and skin rashes. Should be swallowed with water to avoid irritiation to the oesophagus.

Alexitol sodium. Complex of sodium poly(hydroxyaluminium) carbonate and hexitol. An antacid with uses and adverse effects similar to ALUMINIUM HYDROXIDE.

Alfentanil (c). Narcotic analgesic, with actions and uses similar to FENTANYL and MORPHINE. Has a rapid onset of action, but its duration of action is less than other narcotic analgesics. Used as an adjunct to anaesthesia during short surgical procedures.

Alfuzosin. $Alpha_1$ antagonist used for symptomatic relief in benign prostatic hypertrophy. Does not reduce or delay growth of the prostate but reduces urethral tone and resistance and bladder resistance thus relieving the more distressing symptoms. May cause dizziness, headache, gastro-intestinal disturbance, tachycardia, flushing and itching.

Alginic acid. Extract of algae found mainly on the west coast of Scotland and Ireland. Used as tablet binder and disintegrant.

Alimemazine. rINN for TRIMEPRAZINE.

Allantoin. Used in creams and lotions to stimulate wound healing.

Allergen extract vaccines. Extracts prepared from common allergens (e.g., grass, bee venom) for hyposensitization of hypersensitive individuals. Used as graded doses starting from the lowest. Injected subcutaneously. Avoid in pregnancy, febrile conditions and acute asthma. May cause allergic reactions.

Allopurinol. Reduces formation of uric acid from purine precursors by inhibiting the enzyme xanthine oxidase. Used in primary and secondary gout.

Allyloestrenol. Hormone with actions similar to PROGESTERONE.

Almasilate. Polymer of aluminium magnesium silicate. Similar antacid properties to ALUMINIUM HYDROXIDE and MAGNESIUM TRISILICATE.

Aloes. Derived from species of aloe. Used as purgative, producing motion six to twelve hours after ingestion. Causes griping. Colours urine red. May cause nephritis in large doses.

Aloin. Extract of aloes: *see* ALOES.

Aloxiprin. Complex of ALUMINIUM ANTACIDS and ACETYLSALICYLIC ACID, yielding these agents after breakdown in the gastro-intestinal tract.

Alpha-calcidol (1α-Hydroxyvitamin D_3). Rapidly converted in the liver to dihydroxy-vitamin D_3 – the metabolite of vitamin D with the most marked effect on calcium and phosphate balance. Used in treatment of renal bone disease, hypoparathyroidism, rickets, and osteomalacia when these are resistant to vitamin D itself. May cause hypercalcaemia with risk of metastatic calcification and renal failure. Hypercalcaemia treated by stopping the drug and administration of fluids plus potent diuretics (e.g., FRUSEMIDE).

Alphadolone. *See* ALPHAXALONE.

Alphaxalone. Steroid used as intra treatment of anxiety, and anxiety associated with depression.

Alprenolol. Beta-adrenoceptor blocking drug with partial agonist activity (intrinsic sympathomimetic activity). Uses, side effects, etc. as for PROPRANOLOL.

Alprostadil Naturally occurring prostaglandin which increases penile blood flow by direct relaxation of arterial smooth muscle and inhibition of thromboxane. Used by intracavernous (intrapenile) injection in treatment of erectile dysfunction. Adverse effects include burning sensation and pain in the penis. May also cause a fall in blood pressure, cardiac arrhythmias, dizziness and headaches.

Alteplase. A synthetic plasminogen activator/fibrinolytic agent given intravenously after a myocardial infarct to dissolve thrombi in the coronary artery. Unlike STREPTOKINASE and UROKINASE it acts on plasminogen in the clot rather than in the systemic circulation and is not immunogenic. May cause localized bleeding, intracerebral haemorrhage, nausea and vomiting.

Altretamine. Cytotoxic used in treatment of ovarian cancer and other solid dose tumours. May cause bone marrow suppression and gastro-intestinal disturbance.

Alum (Potassium aluminium sulphate). Used as solid to stop bleeding; in powder for application to umbilical cord. Precipitates proteins and is a powerful astringent.

Aluminium antacids. Range of aluminium salts, used alone or complexed with other compounds. Neutralize gastric acid in treatment of peptic ulceration. Large doses cause constipation which may be prevented by combination with MAGNESIUM ANTACIDS. May reduce absorption of other drugs (e.g., TETRACYCLINE).

Aluminium carbonate. Nonsystemic (nonabsorbable) antacid. Used in treatment of peptic ulceration where it produces longer neutralization of acid than SODIUM BICARBONATE. Also used in prevention of urinary phosphate stones. May cause constipation. Reduces absorption of TETRACYCLINE given at same time.

Aluminium chloride. Astringent. Precipitates proteins when applied to skin resulting in hardening and reduced secretions. Used to prevent excessive sweating (hyperhidrosis).

Aluminium chlorohydrate. Used topically in antiperspirant preparations. Thought to act by reducing release of sweat by forming a plug using cell proteins which block the sweat duct. May cause redness or irritation.

Aluminium glycinate. *See* ALUMINIUM ANTACIDS.

Aluminium hydroxide. Nonsystemic (nonabsorbable) antacid. Neutralizes gastric acid and binds phosphate ions in the gut. Used to treat peptic ulceration by reducing gastric acidity and also to increase phosphate excretion when phosphate retention is associated with stone formation (e.g., renal stones). Large doses cause constipation which may be prevented by combination with MAGNESIUM ANTACIDS.

Alverine. Antispasmodic drug used in gut colic; related to PAPAVERINE.

Amantadine. Antiviral agent for prophylaxis against influenza. Antiparkinsonian drug used in mild cases. Adverse effects include dry mouth, visual disturbance, confusion, hallucinations, and ankle oedema.

Ambucetamide. Antispasmodic used in preparations recommended for dysmenorrhoea.

Ambutonium. Anticholinergic with actions similar to ATROPINE SULPHATE. Used in treatment of peptic ulcer.

Amethocaine. Local anaesthetic similar to LIGNOCAINE. Powerful surface activity but toxic by injection. Used topically in ophthalmology.

Amfetamine. rINN for AMPHETAMINE.

Amifostine. Cytoprotective used to reduce the adverse effects of anticancer drugs. It is a prodrug activated by an enzyme which is present in large amounts only where there is a good blood supply. Acts by combining with, and deactivating, the anticancer drug at non-tumour sites, but is less active in most tumours since the blood supply is usually relatively reduced, thus allowing the anticancer drug to exert its effect. Adverse effects include nausea, vomiting, dizziness, and low blood pressure.

Amikacin. Antimicrobial with actions and uses similar to GENTAMICIN.

Amiloride. Potassium-sparing diuretic. Acts by inhibiting exchange of sodium for potassium in the distal tubule of the kidney. Relatively weak diuretic used when there is particular danger of potassium loss (e.g., fluid overload due to liver failure). Often combined with a thiazide (e.g., BENDROFLUAZIDE) or FRUSEMIDE. Danger of excessive potassium retention. May cause nausea, vomiting and diarrhoea.

Aminacrine. Skin disinfectant.

Amino acids. Dietary components. Breakdown products of proteins. Some may be synthesized in the body, others (the 'essential' amino acids) cannot, and must be taken in at least minimum amounts for normal health.

Aminoacridine. *See* AMINACRINE.

Aminobenzoic acid. Member of the vitamin B complex found in some compound vitamin preparations. Used as a lotion to protect the skin from ultraviolet radiation.

Aminoglutethimide. Has inhibitory actions on adrenal cortex. May be used to suppress adrenal activity in hyperadrenalism, particularly when due to adrenal carcinoma. Also used to reduce oedema caused by hyperaldosteronism and in sex hormone dependent prostatic and breast carcinoma. Adverse effects include drowsiness, confusion, skin rashes, gastric discomfort, bone marrow suppression, hypothyroidism, and virilism.

Aminophylline (Theophylline ethylenediamine). Relaxes smooth muscle, dilates bronchi, increases heart rate and force, and has diuretic action. Used in cardiac and bronchial asthma. Given orally, intravenously, or by suppository. Adverse effects include nausea, vomiting, if given orally; vertigo, restlessness, cardiac arrhythmias, if given intravenously.

5-Aminosalicylic acid. *See* MESALAZINE.

Amiodarone. Cardiac antiarrhythmic. Adverse effects include hepatitis, disturbances of thyroid function, corneal deposits, nerve damage, skin photosensitivity, sleep disturbance, and a metallic taste.

Amisulpride. Oral antipsychotic which acts by blocking presynaptic (in low doses) and postsynaptic (at high doses) dopamine receptors (D_2 and D_3). It is thus used to control both the negative and the positive symptoms of schizophrenia. May cause agitation, gastro-intestinal disorders, weight gain and movement disorders.

Amitriptyline. Antidepressant. Actions and adverse effects similar to IMIPRAMINE. Also has sedative and anxiolytic properties.

Amlodipine. Anti-anginal/antihypertensive vasodilator, with actions, uses and adverse effects similar to NIFEDIPINE. Long duration of action allows once daily dosage.

Ammonium chloride. Acidifying agent. Also used as expectorant and diuretic.

Amobarbital. rINN for AMYLOBARBITONE.

Amorolfine. Antifungal agent similar to TERBINAFINE, but marketed as a lacquer for treatment of fungal infections of the nails. May cause pruritus.

Amoxapine. Tricyclic antidepressant which inhibits reuptake of noradrenaline and serotonin in neurones. Adverse effects and precautions as for AMITRIPTYLINE. Said to have a more rapid onset of anti-depressant effects and to be one of the less sedative tricyclics.

Amoxicillin. rINN for AMOXYCILLIN.

Amoxycillin. Similar to AMPICILLIN but better absorbed.

Amphetamine (c). Sympathomimetic amine. Increases heart rate and blood pressure by NORADRENALINE release from sympathetic nerve endings. Produces central stimulation through central noradrenergic and dopaminergic receptor activity. Many uses including as anorectic. Produces dependence and, in prolonged, excessive use, psychosis. Now falling into disuse.

Amphotericin. Antifungal. Used topically for skin infections or by intravenous injection for severe generalized fungal infections. Topically it may produce irritation of skin. Systemic side effects are often severe, including headache, vomiting, fever, joint pains, convulsions, and kidney damage.

Ampicillin. Penicillin antibiotic with broader spectrum of activity than BENZYLPENICILLIN; active against typhoid fever. Adverse effects as for BENZYLPENICILLIN. Rash common if given to patients with infectious mononucleosis (i.e. glandular fever).

Amsacrine. Cytotoxic drug with actions, indications and adverse effects similar to DOXORUBICIN.

Amyl nitrite (m). Vasodilator with actions similar to glyceryl trinitrate but with more rapid onset of action and shorter duration of effect. Abused in the belief that it expands creativity, appreciation of music and sexual experience. Not used to treat angina because adverse effects are accentuated and beneficial actions are too short-lived. Used as an immediate antidote to cyanide poisoning to induce formation of methaemoglobin which combines with cyanide to form non-toxic cyanmethaemoglobin.

Amylobarbitone (c). Barbiturate hypnotic/sedative. General depressant action on CNS. Used in treatment of insomnia and anxiety. Frequently has a 'hangover' effect with impairment of mental and physical performance. Tolerance and addiction may occur, with insomnia, delirium and convulsions on withdrawal. Metabolized by liver and therefore used with caution in liver disease. Induces its own metabolism and that of some other drugs with danger of adverse drug interaction. Coma with respiratory depression in overdosage. No antidote; treated by supportive measures.

Amylocaine. Local anaesthetic with actions similar to LIGNOCAINE.

Anastrozole. Anti-oestrogen, acts by inhibition of an enzyme responsible for production of non-ovarian oestrogens. Breast cancer after the menopause is usually oestrogen-dependent and non-ovarian sources are of increased importance. Used, therefore, to treat advanced breast cancer in post-menopausal women. May cause hot flushes, vaginal irritation, hair thinning, gastro-intestinal disturbance, rash and headaches.

Ancrod. Anticoagulant enzyme from venom of Malayan Pit Viper. Given intravenously. May produce allergic reactions.

Anethole. Essential oil with odour of anise. Used as a carminative and expectorant.

Aneurine (Thiamine, Vitamin B_1). Vitamin. Deficiency may cause cardiac failure (wet beri-beri), peripheral neuritis (dry beri-beri) and Wernicke's encephalopathy.

Angiotensin. Peptide pressor agent given by intravenous infusion in treatment of hypotensive states and shock. Adverse effects include headache and cardiac arrhythmias.

Anistreplase. An acylated complex of human plasminogen with Streptokinase which produces plasmin when injected intravenously and dissolves blood clots. Acylation delays plasmin release. Used after acute myocardial infarction. May produce allergic reactions, treated as for STREPTOKINASE.

Antazoline. Antihistamine with actions and uses similar to PROMETHAZINE.

Anthraquinone glycosides. Derivative of Chinese rhubarb used with SALICYLIC ACID for topical treatment of inflamed and ulcerated conditions in the mouth.

Anti-D immunoglobulin. Human immunoglobulin active against Rhesus (Rh_0D) antibodies. Given to Rhesus negative mothers prophylactically or after delivery of a Rhesus positive child, intended to prevent haemolytic disease of newborn in subsequent pregnancies. May cause anaphylactoid reactions in patients who have antibodies against immunoglobulin A, or who have previously had atypical reactions to blood products.

Antidiuretic hormone. *See* VASOPRESSIN.

Antipyrene. *See* PHENAZONE.

Apomorphine. Stimulates DOPAMINE receptors. Used by injection for treatment of patients with Parkinson's disease resistant to other therapy. Adverse affects similar to those of BROMOCRIPTINE, particularly nausea and vomiting.

Apraclonidine. $Alpha_2$ agonist which reduces secretion of aqueous humour in the anterior chamber of the eye. Used to prevent or reduce intraocular pressure following laser surgery to the eye. May cause lid retraction, blanching of the conjunctiva, dilated pupils and drowsiness.

Aprotinin. Inhibits enzymes that digest proteins. Used in acute pancreatitis. Adverse effects include allergic reactions.

Arachis oil. Extract of ground nut used for nutrition and for softening both faeces and ear wax.

Arginine. Essential amino acid used in treatment of liver coma and in tests of growth hormone secretion.

Ascorbic acid. *See* VITAMIN C.

Aspirin. *See* ACETYLSALICYLIC ACID.

Astemizole. Antihistamine with actions and adverse effects similar to TERFENADINE. May cause serious cardiac arrhythmias in overdosage.

Atenolol. Beta-adrenoceptor blocking drug with limited cardioselectivity. Uses, side effects, etc. as for PROPRANOLOL.

Atorvastatin. Reduces blood levels of cholesterol when diet alone is not effective. Actions and adverse effects similar to SIMVASTATIN.

Atovaquone. Antiprotozoal acts to block nucleic acid synthesis and thus cell growth in certain parasites. Active against the malarial parasite *Pneumocystis carnii*. Used to treat malaria resistant to first-line drugs and to treat *Pneumocystis carnii* pneumonia, a common infective complication in advanced AIDs. May cause rash, nausea, vomiting, diarrhoea, headache, fever and insomnia.

Atracurium. Non-depolarising skeletal muscle relaxant with uses and adverse effects similar to TUBOCURARINE.

Atropine. *See* ATROPINE SULPHATE.

Atropine methonitrate. Anticholinergic with actions, uses, and adverse effects similar to ATROPINE SULPHATE, but has less effect upon CNS and is sometimes considered less toxic.

Atropine sulphate. Parasympatholytic derivative of belladonna plants (e.g., deadly nightshade). Blocks peripheral autonomic cholinergic nerve junctions. Causes dilatation of pupils, paralysis of ocular accommodation, tachycardia, reduced gut motility, decreased secretions, and CNS stimulation. Used intravenously in treatment of bradycardia and anti-cholinesterase poisoning (e.g., due to organophosphorus insecticides), intra-muscularly as part of pre-operative medication, and topically in the eye for optical refraction in children. For parkinsonism and peptic ulceration it has largely been replaced by other anti-cholinergics. May cause dry mouth, blurred vision, glaucoma, and retention of urine. In overdosage, there is tachycardia, fever, flushed skin, dehydration and excitement. Anticholinesterase (e.g., NEOSTIGMINE) may be used as antidote.

Attapulgite. Form of magnesium aluminium silicate used as adsorbent agent in treatment of acute poisoning, in diarrhoea and in topical deodorant preparations.

Auranofin. Orally active gold compound for treatment of rheumatoid arthritis. Actions, uses and adverse effects similar to AUROTHIOMALATE SODIUM.

Aurothiomalate sodium. Preparation of gold for intramuscular injection in treatment of active rheumatoid arthritis. Adverse effects include allergic reactions such as rashes, blood dyscrasias, jaundice, kidney dysfunction, peripheral neuritis, and encephalitis.

Azapropazone. Non-steroid anti-inflammatory/analgesic used in arthritic conditions. Adverse effects include gastro-intestinal disturbances, allergic rashes and photosensitivity. Contra-indicated in patients with a history of peptic ulceration.

Azatadine. Antihistamine with actions, uses, and adverse effects similar to PROMETHAZINE.

Azathioprine. Derivative of MERCAPTOPURINE, used primarily as immunosuppressant agent in patients receiving organ transplants. Adverse effects include bone marrow depression.

Azelaic acid. Antibacterial, anti-inflammatory agent used topically for acne. Prevents growth of the bacteria involved in the development of acne lesions, and reduces the inflammatory response of the white blood cells. Also reduces proliferation of skin cells in the lesions. May cause local skin irritation and photosensitivity.

Azelastine. Antihistamine (H1) nasal spray used for symptomatic relief of allergic rhinitis. By this route the drug does not cause sedation although nasal irritation and taste disturbance may occur.

Azithromycin. Bactericidal antibiotic with spectrum of activity and adverse effects similar to ERYTHROMYCIN, but requires only once daily administration.

Azlocillin. Broad-spectrum antibiotic, with actions and adverse effects similar to CARBENICILLIN.

Aztreonam. Bactericidal antibiotic for injection. May be used cautiously in patients allergic to PENICILLINS and CEPHALOSPORINS. Adverse effects include rashes, diarrhoea, vomiting.

B

Bacampicillin. Pro-drug antibiotic. Readily absorbed from gastro-intestinal tract and rapidly metabolized to the active drug AMPICILLIN, whose actions, uses, and adverse effects it shares.

Bacitracin. Peptide antibiotic active mainly on gram-positive cocci. Nephrotoxic on systemic administration. Only used topically for skin infections.

Baclofen. Used in treatment of skeletal muscle spasticity. Adverse effects include nausea and sedation.

Balsalazide. Prodrug combines MESALAZINE (5-aminosalicylic acid) with an inert carrier. Passes unchanged to the colon where bacterial enzymes release MESALAZINE. Used by mouth in the treatment of ulcerative colitis. May cause headaches and abdominal pain.

Bambuterol. Bronchodilator, pro-drug for TERBUTALINE which improves its availability and prolongs its action. Uses and adverse effects similar to TERBUTALINE.

Beclometasone. rINN for BECLOMETHASONE.

Beclomethasone. Potent synthetic CORTICOSTEROID similar to DEXAMETHASONE. Used by inhalation for treatment of asthma.

Belladonna extract. Plant extract containing ATROPINE SULPHATE and having similar actions, uses, and adverse effects.

Bendrofluazide. Thiazide diuretic used in the treatment of fluid overload and in control of high blood pressure. Acts by reducing sodium reabsorption in the kidney. Less potent than FRUSEMIDE and MERSALYL but has longer action. It is effective orally. May cause excessive loss of potassium in urine and increase in blood uric acid or glucose. Consequently can produce symptoms of hypokalaemia, gout, or diabetes. May produce impotence.

Bendroflumethiazide. rINN for BENDROFLUAZIDE.

Benethamine penicillin. Long-acting form of BENZYLPENICILLIN, with similar actions and adverse effects.

Benorilate. rINN for BENORYLATE.

Benorylate. Analgesic/anti-inflammatory combination that breaks down in the body into ACETYLSALICYLIC ACID and PARACETAMOL, and has the actions of each.

Benoxinate. *See* OXYBUPROCAINE.

Benperidol. Tranquillizer, with actions, uses, etc. similar to HALOPERIDOL.

Benserazide. Used with LEVODOPA in Parkinson's disease. Prevents peripheral breakdown of LEVODOPA, allowing reduced dosage and decreased side effects.

Bentonite. Native colloidal hydrated aluminium silicate used as an adsorbent in treatment of poisoning, and as a pharmaceutical aid in preparation of drug formulations.

Benzalkonium. Topical disinfectant used in creams, lozenges, and irrigating solutions.

Benzathine penicillin. Long-acting form of BENZYLPENICILLIN, with similar actions and adverse effects.

Benzethonium. Similar to BENZALKONIUM.

Benzhexol. Antispasmodic parasympatholytic used in parkinsonism of all causes.

Like ATROPINE, it may produce dry mouth, blurred vision, constipation, hesitancy of micturition, confusion, and hallucinations. Contraindicated in glaucoma and prostate hypertrophy. In overdosage, dry mouth, nausea, vomiting, excitement, confusion, hot dry skin, rapid pulse, and fixed dilated pupils. Depression of respiration and hypotension with loss of consciousness in late stages. Salicylate of PHYSOSTIGMINE is effective antidote.

Benzilonium. Parasympatholytic with peripheral effects, toxic effects, etc. similar to ATROPINE SULPHATE. Used as antispasmodic for gastro-intestinal disorders and to reduce gastric acid secretion in peptic ulceration.

Benzocaine. Weak local anaesthetic similar to LIGNOCAINE. Used in proprietary preparations for sore throats.

Benzoctamine. Anxiolytic. Actions, uses and adverse effects similar to DIAZEPAM.

Benzoic acid. Used topically for mild fungus infections of skin.

Benzoin. Plant resin extract used as inhalation to reduce catarrh in upper respiratory tract and as topical skin preparation to reduce or prevent dryness and fissures.

Benzoylmetronidazole. Antibacterial, formulated as suspension for those unable to swallow tablets. Otherwise identical to METRONIDAZOLE.

Benzoyl peroxide. Antiseptic/keratolytic. Powder used in dusting powders and in creams and lotions in treatment of burns, skin ulcers, and acne.

Benzthiazide. Diuretic, with actions similar to CHLOROTHIAZIDE.

Benztropine. Antispasmodic parasympatholytic used in parkinsonism. Similar to BENZHEXOL, but more potent and can be given by intramuscular injection. Particularly useful in treating drug-induced parkinsonism.

Benzydamine. Analgesic with anti-inflammatory and antipyretic properties similar to ACETYLSALICYLIC ACID. Used topically as cream for musculoskeletal pains and as a mouthwash for sore throat. Overdosage by mouth has caused agitation, anxiety, hallucinations, and convulsions.

Benzyl benzoate. Used as insect repellent, in treatment of scabies, and as antipruritic. May cause allergic rashes.

Benzyl nicotinate. Vasodilator related to NICOTINIC ACID.

Benzylpenicillin. Bactericidal antibiotic (*see* PENICILLINS). Unstable at acid pH, poorly active by mouth. Given parenterally. Active against most gram-positive and some gram-negative organisms. Inactivated by penicillinase. Adverse effects include hypersensitivity reactions, both immediate and delayed, and encephalopathy with convulsions if given intrathecally or in massive doses.

Bephenium. Used in treatment of hookworms. Adverse effects include nausea, vomiting, and vertigo.

Beractant. A synthetic surfactant used to treat lung damage (Respiratory Distress Syndrome) in preterm infants. Similar to COLFOSCERIL.

Betahistine. Vasodilator with actions similar to HISTAMINE. Used in Ménière's disease to reduce episodes of dizziness.

Betamethasone. Potent synthetic CORTICOSTEROID similar to DEXAMETHASONE.

Betanidine. rINN for BETHANIDINE.

Betaxolol. Beta-adrenoceptor blocking drug with cardioselectivity. Used as an antihypertensive, and as eye drops for glaucoma. Adverse effects and precautions as for PROPRANOLOL.

Betazole. Related to HISTAMINE, with similar actions and uses.

Bethanechol. Parasympathomimetic drug, with actions of ACETYLCHOLINE.

Bethanidine. Adrenergic neurone blocking drug. Used in hypertension. Adverse effects as for GUANETHIDINE.

Bezafibrate. Reduces blood fats, with uses, interactions, and adverse effects similar to CLOFIBRATE.

Bicalutamide. Antiandrogen used in the treatment of cancer of the prostate. May cause hot flushes, itching, breast enlargement/tenderness and angina.

Bile salts. Extracted from animal bile. Used to stimulate bile flow without increasing its bile salts and pigment contents (e.g., after biliary operations). Included in some compound preparations for treatment of biliary insufficiency, but of doubtful efficacy.

Biotin (Vitamin H). Found in liver, kidney, yeast, eggs, and milk. Until recently there was no known clinical deficiency state. Induced deficiency caused dermatitis, lassitude, anorexia, and parasthesiae. It is now known that several extremely rare inborn metabolic disorders present with similar symptoms and respond to biotin.

Biperiden. Parasympatholytic antispasmodic used in treatment of parkinsonism of all causes. Actions and adverse effects similar to BENZHEXOL but may also cause drowsiness. Overdose effects similar to BENZHEXOL.

Bisacodyl. Purgative that acts by stimulating sensory nerve endings in wall of large bowel. Available for oral and rectal use. Suppositories may cause mild burning sensation in the rectum.

Bismuth aluminate. *See* BISMUTH ANTACIDS.

Bismuth antacids. Insoluble bismuth salts have weak antacid properties and are claimed to protect the stomach. Largely superseded by more effective antacids. Prolonged, excessive use may allow sufficient absorption to cause toxicity with kidney damage, liver damage, and CNS effects.

Bismuth carbonate. *See* BISMUTH ANTACIDS.

Bismuth chelate. *See* TRI-POTASSIUM DICITRATO BISMUTHATE.

Bismuth oxide. *See* BISMUTH ANTACIDS.

Bismuth salicylate. Bismuth salt administered by mouth for protective effect on stomach and bowels. Converted to bismuth and SODIUM SALICYLATE in small intestine. Used as symptomatic treatment for indigestion, nausea, and diarrhoea.

Bismuth subgallate. Insoluble powder used for eczema and as suppositories for haemorrhoids.

Bismuth subnitrate. *See* BISMUTH ANTACIDS.

Bisoprolol. Cardioselective beta-adrenoceptor blocking drug. Used in the treatment of hypertension and angina. Actions and adverse effects similar to ATENOLOL.

Bleomycin. Cytotoxic antibiotic used to treat lymphomas and solid tumours. Toxic effects include lung fibrosis and skin pigmentation.

Boric acid. Weak anti-infective powder used in dusting powders, lotions, and ointments.

Botulinum toxin A. Neurotoxin derived from the bacterium *Clostridium botulinum.* Binds to endings of nerves which supply muscles, to prevent the release of ACETYLCHOLINE, so producing weakness or paralysis of those muscles, from which recovery occurs after 2–3 months. Used by local injection to treat patients with troublesome spasm of the eyelids, strabismus (squint) and twitching of muscles around the mouth. Effects seen within 2–5 days of injection. Unwanted effects include bruising around the eye, double vision, drooping eyelid, and weakness of facial muscles.

Bran. Purgative, non-irritant. Byproduct of milling of wheat. Contains indigestible cellulose which increases intestinal bulk. Crude bran is unpalatable; processed bran is pleasant cereal. Large doses needed for effect. Danger of bowel obstruction if pre-existing bowel narrowing.

Bretylium. Adrenergic neurone blocking drug with actions similar to GUANETHIDINE. Used mainly in cardiac arrhythmias. Side effects have limited its use as anti-hypertensive.

Brimonidine. Selective alpha adrenoceptor blocking agent used topically in the treatment of glaucoma. Less likely to produce systemic central nervous system or cardiac effects than some other glaucoma treatments. May cause local irritation, allergic reactions and drowsiness. Acts by reducing formation of aqueous humour and improving drainage.

Bromazepam. Benzodiazepine anxiolytic, with actions and adverse effects similar to DIAZEPAM.

Bromides. CNS depressants, now largely superseded by safer drugs.

Bromocriptine. Stimulates dopamine receptors. Used in treatment of acromegaly, for inhibition or suppression of lactation, and in conditions due to excessive prolactin secretion, including some cases of infertility and in some patients with Parkinson's disease. Adverse effects include nausea, hypotension, and cold extremities.

Brompheniramine. Antihistamine, with actions similar to PROMETHAZINE.

Bronopol. Antibacterial preservative used in topical preparations.

Buclizine. Antihistamine/anti-emetic drug with actions similar to PROMETHAZINE.

Budesonide. Synthetic CORTICOSTEROID similar to DEXAMETHASONE. Used by inhalation for treatment of asthma. Also applied intranasally for allergic rhinitis, and topically for psoriasis and eczema and systemically in a controlled release form for Crohn's disease.

Bumetanide. Potent diuretic, with actions and uses similar to FRUSEMIDE. Adverse effects similar to BENDROFLUAZIDE.

Bupivacaine. Local anaesthetic similar to LIGNOCAINE, but produces longer anaesthesia.

Buprenorphine (c). Narcotic analgesic with antagonist properties for injection or as sublingual tablets. Actions, uses, and adverse effects similar to PENTAZOCINE.

Buserelin. Hormone. Analogue of gonadotrophin-releasing hormone that suppresses androgen production by testes. Used in treatment of carcinoma of the prostate and endometriosis. May cause hot flushes, nasal irritation and loss of libido.

Buspirone. Anxiolytic used in short-term relief of the symptoms of anxiety. Acts by different (but, as yet, undefined) mechanisms to the benzodiazepines. Does not have muscle relaxant or anticonvulsant effects. Takes longer to have an effect than the benzodiazepines, but appears to cause less sedation and is less likely to lead to dependence. May cause headaches and dizziness.

Busulfan. rINN for BUSULPHAN.

Busulphan. Cytotoxic drug used in neoplastic disease, particularly myeloid leukaemia. Adverse effects include skin pigmentation, cataract, pulmonary fibrosis, and bone marrow depression.

Butacaine. Local anaesthetic used by injection or by spray on to the mucosa of the nose and throat. Actions and adverse effects similar to LIGNOCAINE.

Butethamate. Sympathomimetic amine, with actions similar to EPHEDRINE.

Butobarbital. rINN for BUTOBARBITONE.

Butobarbitone (c). Barbiturate hypnotic essentially like AMYLOBARBITONE.

Butorphanol (d). Analgesic injection, with actions and uses similar to MORPHINE, but has narcotic antagonist activity similar to NALOXONE. May cause sedation, dizziness, nausea, changes in mood, and vivid dreams. Has low potential for dependence and addiction, and may precipitate withdrawal symptoms in narcotic addicts. May depress respiration and therefore caution is advised if used in patients with respiratory disease. NALOXONE, but not NALORPHINE or LEVALLORPHAN, may be used as antagonist.

Butoxyethyl nicotinate. *See* NICOTINIC ACID.

Butriptyline. Antidepressant, with actions and uses similar to IMIPRAMINE.

Butyl nitrite (m). Vasodilator with actions, adverse effects and abuse potential similar to amyl nitrite.

C

Cabergoline. Ergot derivative with dopamine agonist activity. A prolactin antagonist similar to BROMOCRIPTINE but with less risk of cardiac toxicity at recommended doses. Used after pregnancy to -suppress unwanted lactation and to facilitate conception when infertility is associated with high prolactin levels. Also used to control symptoms of Parkinson's disease.

Caffeine. Active principle from tea and coffee, used as mild CNS stimulant. Adverse effects include restlessness, excitement, and dependence after prolonged excessive ingestion. Claimed to enhance the absorption and thus the effectiveness of ERGOTAMINE in migraine.

Calamine. Zinc carbonate used in dusting powders, creams, lotions, etc.

Calciferol. *See* VITAMIN D.

Calcipotriol. Synthetic analogue of VITAMIN D used topically as treatment for psoriasis. Acts on vitamin D receptors in skin cells (keratocytes) to reduce cell proliferation and thus corrects one of the key abnormalities in that condition. Unlike CALCITRIOL (natural vitamin D3) this drug has little effect on calcium metabolism thus reducing the risk of hypercalcaemia. May cause local irritation.

Calcitonin. rINN for SALCATONIN.

Calcitriol. (1α,25-Dihydroxycholecalciferol). More potent active metabolite of VITAMIN D. Used intravenously in dialysis patients to treat/prevent hypocalcaemia and renal bone disease and orally to treat postmenopausal osteoporosis.

Calcium carbonate. Nonsystemic (non-absorbable) antacid. Used in treatment of peptic ulceration where it produces longer neutralization of acid than SODIUM BICARBONATE. Frequent use may cause constipation. Small amounts are absorbed and in some subjects may cause renal stones (i.e. nephrocalcinosis). When formulated as an effervescent tablet, yields CALCIUM CITRATE in the stomach.

Calcium chloride. Used intravenously as a source of calcium ions in treatment of cardiac arrest. Orally, could be used as a dietary supplement, but is very irritant to the gastro-intestinal tract. CALCIUM GLUCONATE or CALCIUM PHOSPHATE are preferred for this purpose.

Calcium citrate. Absorbable calcium salt used as a calcium supplement in deficiency states and in osteoporosis. Adverse effects include gastro-intestinal disturbance, bone pain, thirst, increased urine output, muscle weakness and confusion.

Calcium gluconate. Source of calcium for deficiency states.

Calcium hydrogen phosphate. Source of calcium and phosphate for treatment of dietary insufficiency.

Calcium iodide. Used as expectorant.

Calcium lactate. *See* CALCIUM GLUCONATE.

Calcium laevulinate. Source of calcium for treatment of dietary insufficiency.

Calcium pantothenate. Source of PANTOTHENIC ACID. Considered a vitamin but no proven deficiency has been discovered.

No accepted therapeutic role, but used in some vitamin mixtures.

Calcium phosphate. Source of calcium for treatment of dietary insufficiency.

Calcium polystyrene sulphonate. Ion exchange resin used to treat electrolyte abnormalities by changing absorption or excretion in the gut.

Calcium sulphaloxate. Sulphonamide antibacterial, with actions similar to SULPHADIMIDINE. Very little absorbed. Used for prevention or treatment of mild infective diarrhoea.

Camphene. *See* CAMPHOR.

Camphor. Used internally as carminative and externally as rubefacient.

Candesartan cilexetil. Prodrug, rapidly absorbed and converted to candesartan ANGIOTENSIN II receptor antagonist with actions, uses and adverse effects similar to LOSARTAN.

Candicidin. Antifungal antibiotic used locally for vaginal and skin infections.

Cannabis (m). Dried extract of the plant *Cannabis sativa*, smoked or taken by mouth for the promotion of mood elevation. The main active principle is tetrahydrocannabinol. Adverse effects include nausea, vomiting, anxiety and psychotic episodes. Tolerance and psychological dependence occur but physical dependence is not a serious problem. Overdose causes exacerbation of the adverse effects and is managed by supportive treatment. Cannabinoids have antiemetic effects. NABILONE is a cannabis derivative used to treat nausea and vomiting from cytotoxic drugs.

Capreomycin. Peptide antibiotic, mainly used in tuberculosis. Adverse effects include ototoxicity and nephrotoxicity.

Capsaicin. Naturally occurring substance found in *Capsicum* (sweet pepper). When applied to the skin it depletes local pain-conducting nerve fibres of pain transmitter substance. Used topically to treat post-herpetic neuralgia (pain persisting after shingles, which is caused by infection with the herpes zoster virus). Claimed to be effective in treating pain after Psoralin Ultra Violet Activation therapy and in erythromelalgia. Should not be applied to broken skin. May cause skin irritation.

Capsicum. Essential oil used internally as carminative and externally as rubefacient.

Captopril. Inhibits angiotensin-converting enzyme (ACE) involved in formation of hormone concerned with maintenance of blood pressure and constriction of blood vessels. Used in treatment of hypertension, kidney disease in diabetic patients, chronic heart failure and in prevention of recurrent myocardial infarction. Adverse effects include hypotension, proteinuria and renal impairment, skin rashes and cough. Bone marrow depression and loss of taste may occur with high doses.

Caraway. Essential oil used as carminative.

Carbachol. Parasympathomimetic, with actions and adverse effects similar to ACETYLCHOLINE, but more prolonged. Used as miotic eye drops in glaucoma and for improvement of postoperative intestinal or bladder muscle tone.

Carbamazepine. Anticonvulsant. Acts by suppressing epileptic discharges in the brain. Used in prevention of epilepsy, in suppression of pain in trigeminal neuralgia (but is not an analgesic), and in mania. May cause drowsiness, blurred vision, dizziness, and gastro-intestinal upsets. Skin rashes and adverse effects on the liver and bone marrow are relatively common. Coma with convulsions in overdosage. No antidote; supportive treatment only.

Carbaryl. Anticholinesterase. Used topically as an insecticide (e.g. for lice).

Carbenicillin. PENICILLIN antibiotic, particularly active against gram-negative bacteria especially *Pseudomonas* and *Proteus*. Adverse effects as for BENZYLPENICILLIN.

Carbenoxolone. Used in treatment of gastric and duodenal ulcers and for mouth ulcers. Has ALDOSTERONE-like actions. Adverse effects include oedema, hypertension, hypokalaemia, and muscle pain.

Carbidopa. Similar actions to BENSERAZIDE.

Carbimazole. Depresses formation of thyroid hormone. Used in treatment of hyperthyroidism. Adverse effects include allergic rashes, nausea, diarrhoea, blood abnormalities, and keratitis.

Carbinoxamine. Antihistamine, with actions similar to PROMETHAZINE.

Carbocysteine. Mucolytic used to reduce viscosity of sputum.

Carboplatin. Cytotoxic with actions, uses and adverse effects similar to CISPLATIN.

Carboprost. Synthetic prostaglandin used in treatment of post-partum haemorrhage which fails to respond to OXYTOCIN or SYNTOCIN/ERGOMETRINE. Adverse effects include gastro-intestinal disturbances, hyperthermia, flushing, asthma, hypertension, dyspnoea, and pulmonary oedema.

Carisoprodol. Used to treat painful muscle spasm.

Carmellose. Cellulose derivative employed in artificial tears and as a pharmaceutical aid in drug formulations.

Carmustine. Intravenous cytotoxic, inactivates DNA, RNA, and several enzymes. Crosses the blood-brain barrier, thus useful for brain tumours as well as certain other neoplastic diseases. Rapidly degraded from the parent drug to active metabolites. Adverse effects include nausea, vomiting, burning sensation at injection site, renal and hepatic damage, and delayed bone marrow suppression.

Carteolol. Beta-adrenoceptor blocking drug used in prevention of angina. Actions and adverse effects similar to PROPRANOLOL.

Carvedilol. Non-selective beta adrenoceptor antagonist with alpha antagonist activity. Used as prophylaxis of stable angina and in treatment of hypertension where its effects and adverse effects are similar to LABETALOL.

Cascara. Purgative from bark of buckthorn tree. Stimulates gut movement via the nerve plexus in the large bowel wall. Produces reddish-brown discoloration of urine and may cause excessive catharsis. Excreted in milk of lactating mothers and may cause diarrhoea in infants. Prolonged use causes black pigmentation in colon (melanosis coli).

Castor oil. Purgative, with action upon small intestine as well as large intestine useful when prompt evacuation is required (e.g., before bowel X-rays). Chronic use not recommended as it causes reduced absorption of nutrients. Also used topically on skin for its emollient effect.

Cefaclor. CEPHALOSPORIN antibiotic.Orally active and has wider range of activity than earlier drugs of that group. Actions, uses, and adverse effects similar to CEPHALOTHIN.

Cefadroxil. CEPHALOSPORIN antibiotic similar to CEPHALEXIN.

Cefalexin. rINN for CEPHALEXIN.

Cefamandole. rINN for CEPHAMANDOLE.

Cefazolin. rINN for CEPHAZOLIN.

Cefixime. Cephalosporin antibiotic with wide range of activity. Adverse effects include gastro-intestinal disturbances, headache, dizziness and skin reactions.

Cefotaxime. Broad-spectrum CEPHALOSPORIN antibiotic for injection, with actions, uses, and adverse effects similar to CEPHALOTHIN.

Cefoxitin. Cephamycin antibiotic for injection. Related to the CEPHALOSPORINS with similar actions, uses, and adverse effects, but may have broader spectrum of activity.

Cefpirome. Broad spectrum CEPHALOSPORIN antibiotic which is active against beta-lactamase producing bacteria. Uses and adverse effects similar to other CEPHALOSPORIN antibiotics.

Cefpodoxime proxetil. CEPHALOSPORIN antibiotic, administered orally as its proxetil ester, which is hydrolysed in the gut wall to produce the active drug. Has a broad spectrum of antibacterial activity. Adverse effects include gastro-intestinal and allergic reactions.

Cefradine. rINN for CEPHRADINE.

Cefsoludin. Injectable CEPHALOSPORIN antibiotic with narrow spectrum but specifically active against *Pseudomonas aeruginosa* infections. Dosage must be reduced in renal failure since this drug is excreted unchanged in the urine. Other adverse effects as for CEPHALOTHIN.

Ceftazidime. CEPHALOSPORIN antibiotic used orally and by injection. Has wider range of antibacterial activity than earlier drugs of this group. Adverse effects similar to CEPHALOTHIN.

Ceftibuten. Orally active CEPHALOSPORIN antibiotic. Adverse reactions include gastro-intestinal disturbance, headache and rash.

Ceftizoxime. CEPHALOSPORIN antibiotic for injection. Has range of antibacterial activity similar to CEFTAZIDIME. Adverse effects similar to CEPHALOTHIN.

Ceftriaxone. Broad spectrum CEPHALOSPORIN antibiotic for injection, with actions, uses and adverse effects similar to CEPHALOTHIN.

Cefuroxime. CEPHALOSPORIN antibiotic used orally and by injection. Has wider range of antibacterial activity than earlier drugs in this group. Actions, uses, and adverse effects similar to CEPHALOTHIN.

Celiprolol. Cardioselective beta adrenoceptor-blocking drug with actions and adverse effects similar to ATENOLOL/ACEBUTOLOL. Used to treat hypertension.

Cephalexin. CEPHALOSPORIN antibiotic, with similar activity and adverse effects to CEPHALOTHIN, but well absorbed by mouth.

Cephaloridine. CEPHALOSPORIN antibiotic, administered parenterally. May cause renal damage, particularly if given with FRUSEMIDE. Other adverse effects include hypersensitivity reactions.

Cephalosporins. Bactericidal antibiotics that inhibit bacterial cell wall synthesis. Have similar basic structure to PENICILLINS, but are relatively resistant to penicillinase. Among this drug group, CEPHALORIDINE alone has been clearly implicated as a cause of renal damage.

Cephalothin. CEPHALOSPORIN antibiotic, particularly useful against penicillinase-producing *Staphylococcus aureus*. Must be given parenterally. Adverse effects mainly hypersensitivity reactions.

Cephamandole. Newer CEPHALOSPORIN antibiotic for injection. Has wider range of antibacterial activity than earlier drugs of this group. Actions, uses, and adverse effects similar to CEPHALOTHIN.

Cephazolin. CEPHALOSPORIN antibiotic similar to CEPHALEXIN.

Cephradine. CEPHALOSPORIN antibiotic similar to CEPHALEXIN.

Ceratonia. Powder prepared from the endosperm of the locust bean tree (*Ceratonia siliqua*). Used as a mucilage to thicken feeds for children with diarrhoea.

Cerivastatin. Enzyme inhibitor active in reducing cholesterol synthesis with actions and uses similar to SIMVASTATIN. Adverse effects include headache, rhinitis, cough, influenza-like symptoms, arthralgia, myalgia, back pain, abdominal pain and insomnia.

Certoparin. Anticoagulant, low molecular heparin similar to ENOXAPARIN.

Cetalkonium. Topical disinfectant.

Cetirizine dihydrochloride. Antihistamine used for hay fever and allergic skin conditions. It is rapidly absorbed and has a long duration of action suitable for once-daily dosing. It is related to HYDROXYZINE, but produces less sedation and only mild side effects, including headache, dizziness agitation, dry mouth and gastro-intestinal upset.

Cetomacrogol. Emulsifying wax used in formulating oil-in-water emulsions.

Cetostearyl alcohol. Mixture of solid alcohols used for emulsifying properties in oil-in-water formulations including preparations for protection of dry skin.

Cetrimide. Topical disinfectant used in many skin preparations.

Cetyl alcohol. Used in manufacture of ointments and creams.

Cetylpyridinium. Topical disinfectant used in skin and mouth preparations.

Chamomile oil. An ESSENTIAL OIL used to treat early stages of skin inflammation e.g. nappy rash, cracked nipples. Contact sensitivity has been described.

Charcoal. Used as adsorbent in first aid treatment of poisoning by drugs and toxins. Also used to treat diarrhoea.

Chenodeoxycholic acid. Naturally occurring bile acid which prevents formation and aids dissolution of gall stones.

Chloral betaine. Complex of CHLORAL HYDRATE and trimethyl glycine. Rapidly broken down in the body to yield CHLORAL HYDRATE.

Chloral hydrate. Hypnotic. Available only as a liquid. Converted by liver to trichloroethanol which causes generalized CNS depression. Used for insomnia, especially in children and the elderly. Relatively 'safe'. Addiction is rare. Coma in overdosage. No antidote; treated by supportive measures.

Chlorambucil. Cytotoxic drug related to MUSTINE HYDROCHLORIDE. Used in neoplastic conditions of lymphoid tissues. Adverse effects include bone marrow depression.

Chloramphenicol. Broad-spectrum bacteriostatic antibiotic, which should be reserved for treatment of typhoid fever and life-threatening infections. Adverse effects include aplastic anaemia. Produces 'grey baby syndrome' in neonates and premature babies.

Chlorbutol. Antibacterial and antifungal preservative for topical applications.

Chlorcyclizine. Antihistamine, with similar actions and adverse effects to PROMETHAZINE. Used mainly as an antiemetic.

Chlordantoin. Topical antifungal agent.

Chlordiazepoxide (m). Benzodiazepine anxiolytic similar to DIAZEPAM but less hypnotic and less anticonvulsant activity. Used in treatment of anxiety.

Chlorexolone. Diuretic, with actions, uses, and adverse effects similar to BENDROFLUAZIDE.

Chlorhexidine. Topical disinfectant used in skin preparations, urethral catheterization, cytoscopy, and as preservative in eye drops.

Chlormethiazole. Sedative/hypnotic/anticonvulsant. Depressant action on CNS. Used for sedation or hypnosis in agitated or confused patients especially the elderly. Also for treatment of acute withdrawal symptoms in alcoholics and drug addicts and control of sustained epileptic fits (status epilepticus). May cause tingling in nose and sneezing. Effects potentiated by CHLORPROMAZINE, HALOPERIDOL and related drugs. Coma with respiratory depression in overdosage. No antidote. Symptomatic treatment is adequate.

Chlormethine. rINN for MUSTINE.

Chlormezanone. Anxiolytic, muscle relaxant. Sometimes used as a hypnotic. Actions similar to MEPROBAMATE. Adverse effects include drowsiness, dizziness, headache, skin rashes and jaundice.

Chlorobutanol. rINN for CHLORBUTOL.

Chlorocresol. Disinfectant used in sterilizing solutions and as a preservative in creams.

Chlorofluoromethane. Aerosol propellant for drugs administered by inhalation. Also used as a spray for muscle pain where it produces local anaesthesia due to intense coldness.

Chlorophenoxyethanol. Topical antibacterial.

Chloroquine. Antimalarial agent, which has also been used in rheumatoid arthritis. Adverse effects include skin pigmentation, alopecia, neuropathy, and corneal and retinal damage.

Chlorothiazide. Thiazide diuretic similar to BENDROFLUAZIDE.

Chlorotrianisene. Synthetic female sex hormone used in menopausal symptoms and to suppress lactation. Adverse effects similar to OESTRADIOL.

Chloroxylenol. Topical disinfectant used chiefly on skin.

Chlorphenamine. rINN for CHLORPHENIRAMINE.

Chlorphenesin. Topical antibacterial/antifungal agent.

Chlorpheniramine. Antihistamine, with actions, uses, and adverse effects similar to PROMETHAZINE.

Chlorphenoxamine. Antihistamine similar to PROMETHAZINE used in Parkinson's disease.

Chlorphentermine (c). Anorectic, sympathomimetic amine. Actions and adverse effects similar to DIETHYLPROPION.

Chlorpromazine. Phenothiazine tranquillizer. Causes selective depression of the brain structures responsible for control of behaviour and wakefulness. Has anticholinergic alpha-adrenergic blocking and dopaminergic effects amongst other pharmacological effects. Used in psychotic disorders, particularly schizophrenia and agitated depression; in terminal illness to enhance analgesia; to control nausea and vomiting; and for hiccups. Adverse effects include postural hypotension, dry mouth, blurred vision, involuntary movements, cholestatic jaundice, photosensitivity, and deposits in lens and cornea. Used only with caution in liver disease and epilepsy (may precipitate convulsions). In overdosage causes coma, involuntary movements, convulsions, hypotension, and arrhythmias. No antidote; supportive treatment only.

Chlorpropamide. Oral antidiabetic drug that stimulates pancreatic insulin release in maturity-onset diabetes mellitus. Adverse effects include hypoglycaemia, allergic reactions, jaundice, and flushing with alcohol. Action may be potentiated by salicylates and sulphonamides. Sometimes used in diabetes insipidus.

Chlorprothixene. Phenothiazine tranquillizer essentially similar to CHLORPROMAZINE.

Chlorquinaldol. Topical antibacterial/antifungal similar to HYDROXYQUINOLINE. Used in skin infections.

Chlortalidone. rINN for CHLORTHALIDONE.

Chlortetracycline. Bacteriostatic antibiotic, with actions, adverse effects, and interactions similar to TETRACYCLINE.

Chlorthalidone. Diuretic essentially similar to BENDROFLUAZIDE.

Cholecalciferol. Naturally occurring form of VITAMIN D.

Cholesterol. Natural fatty constituent of all animal cells and a precursor of steroids. Used topically in creams for soothing and water-absorbing properties.

Cholestyramine. Resin that binds bile salts in gut. Used in pruritus associated with jaundice and to reduce blood cholesterol. Adverse effects include nausea, diarrhoea, and constipation.

Choline magnesium trisalicylate. A mixture of CHOLINE SALICYLATE and magnesium salicylate with actions, uses, and adverse effects similar to ACETYLSALICYLIC ACID.

Choline salicylate. Similar actions to ACETYLSALICYLIC ACID.

Choline theophyllinate. Oral preparation of THEOPHYLLINE, with actions similar to AMINOPHYLLINE. Main use is in chronic bronchitis.

Chorionic gonadotrophin. Hormone produced in the placenta. Used in treatment of anovulatory infertility and failure of development of the testes or ovaries. May cause fluid retention and therefore used with caution if there is evidence of cardiac or renal failure.

Chymotrypsin. Animal pancreatic enzyme used to reduce soft tissue inflammation, particularly associated with trauma. Adverse effects include allergic reactions.

Cidofovir. Antiviral agent active against cytomegalovirus, which may be a cause of serious infection in immunocompromised patients, especially those with AIDS.

Cilastatin. Structurally similar to the antibiotic IMIPENEM, but has no antibacterial activity. Given with IMIPENEM it reduces the metabolism of the latter and prolongs its effectiveness. For adverse effects *see* IMIPENEM.

Cilazapril. Pro-drug ACE inhibitor metabolized to the active drug cilazaprilat. Used to treat hypertension. Actions and adverse effects similar to CAPTOPRIL.

Cimetidine. Selectively blocks histamine receptors mediating gastric acid secretion. Used in peptic ulceration and gastric hyperacidity, oesophageal reflux and prophylaxis of gastro-intestinal bleeding in seriously ill patients. Adverse effects include diarrhoea, dizziness, rash and breast enlargement in males. Danger of CNS depression and confusional states in renal failure, the elderly, or seriously ill patients. Increases effects of some other drugs including WARFARIN and PHENYTOIN by reducing their metabolism and excretion.

Cinchocaine. Local anaesthetic with actions similar to LIGNOCAINE.

Cinnarizine. Antihistamine similar to PROMETHAZINE, chiefly used in treatment of vertigo and vomiting.

Cinoxacin. Antibacterial for urinary infections. Actions and adverse effects similar to NALIDIXIC ACID.

Ciprofibrate. Lipid-lowering drug. Acts by reducing cholesterol synthesis and increasing breakdown of lipids. Used to treat hyperlipidaemias not responding to treatment with diet alone. May cause headache, dizziness, drowsiness, rash, muscle pains and gastro-intestinal disturbance .

Ciprofloxacin. Broad-spectrum antibiotic used in a wide range of infections, notably urinary and respiratory, where the organisms are resistant to PENICILLINS and CEPHALOSPORINS. Also used topically for conjunctivitis. Causes bacterial death whether or not the bacteria are growing. Adverse effects include rashes, gastro-intestinal disturbance, headaches, dizziness, tiredness, tendon damage and, if injected, pain at the injection site. Structure similar to NALIDIXIC ACID.

Cisapride. A prokinetic agent related to METOCLOPRAMIDE which facilitates movement throughout the gastrointestinal tract. Used to treat symptoms and lesions of gastro-oesophageal reflux and relieve symptoms of delayed gastric emptying. May cause abdominal cramps and diarrhoea but unlike METOCLOPRAMIDE is not associated with involuntary movements.

Cisatracurium. Non-depolarising muscle relaxant with an intermediate duration of action. Used in surgery and intensive care. Mechanism of action similar to TUBOCURARINE, but without significant adverse effects on blood pressure.

Cisplatin. Cytotoxic platinum compound used in treatment of metastatic testicular and ovarian tumours. May cause renal damage, ototoxicity, bone marrow suppression, nausea, vomiting and allergic reactions.

Citalopram. Antidepressant with actions, uses and adverse effects similar to FLUVOXAMINE.

Cladribine. Cytotoxic with specific effects in hairy cell leukaemia. Adverse effects include bone marrow suppression, renal and neurotoxicity. May also cause gastro-intestinal disturbance and painful reactions at injection sites.

Clarithromycin. Bactericidal antibiotic with spectrum of activity similar to ERYTHROMYCIN, but requires only twice daily administration and unwanted gastro-intestinal effects appear to be less frequent.

Clavulanic acid. Inhibits the enzyme penicillinase which inactivates penicillin antibiotics. Used with AMOXYCILLIN to increase its spectrum of activity. Rare side effects include severe liver toxicity.

Clemastine. Antihistamine, with actions and uses similar to PROMETHAZINE, but with less sedative effects.

Clemizole. Antihistamine similar to PROMETHAZINE.

Clindamycin. Antibiotic, with actions and adverse effects similar to LINCOMYCIN, but better absorbed.

Clioquinol. Used in treatment of gut amoebiasis and to protect against gut infections, used topically for skin infections. Prolonged large oral doses may produce neuropathy.

Clobazam. Benzodiazepine anxiolytic with actions, uses, and adverse effects similar to DIAZEPAM. May also be used for long-term anticonvulsant therapy, similar to CLONAZEPAM.

Clobetasol. Topical CORTICOSTEROID for psoriasis and eczema.

Clobetasone. Topical CORTICOSTEROID for psoriasis and eczema.

Clofazimine. Antileprotic/anti-inflammatory, used for control of reactions occurring with DAPSONE treatment. Adverse effects include skin pigmentation, red urine, and diarrhoea.

Clofibrate. Reduces blood cholesterol and fats. Used in patients with raised levels of these constituents. Adverse effects include nausea, diarrhoea, muscle pain, and weakness. Potentiates anticoagulants.

Clomethiazole. rINN for CHLORMETHIAZOLE.

Clomifene. rINN for CLOMIPHENE.

Clomiphene. Sex hormone used in infertility due to failure of ovulation. Acts both on the pituitary gonadotrophic hormones and on the ovary permitting ovulation. Should not be used in liver failure or if patient has ovarian cysts. Danger of multiple births, especially at higher doses.

Clomipramine. Antidepressant drug, with actions and uses similar to IMIPRAMINE.

Clomocycline. Bacteriostatic antibiotic, with actions, adverse effects, and interactions similar to TETRACYCLINE.

Clonazepam. Benzodiazepine anticonvulsant similar to DIAZEPAM but has greater anticonvulsant activity. Used intravenously for control of status epilepticus, orally for prevention of all types of epilepsy.

Clonidine. Reduces sympathetic activity by central action, and reduces vascular reactivity. Used in hypertension and in migraine. Antihypertensive effect blocked by tricyclic antidepressants. Adverse effects include sedation, depression, dryness of mouth, fluid retention. Rapid withdrawal may be associated with 'rebound hypertension'.

Clopamide. Diuretic essentially similar to BENDROFLUAZIDE.

Clopenthixol. Major tranquillizer with actions similar to CHLORPROMAZINE. Used in treatment of schizophrenia. Sedation and hypotension are predictable adverse effects. Extrapyramidal (parkinsonian) symptoms are less frequent than with CHLORPROMAZINE.

Cloral betaine. rINN for CHLORAL BETAINE.

Clorazepate. Anxiolytic, with actions, uses, and adverse effects similar to DIAZEPAM. Long-acting and has sedative effects, so is best given at night. Metabolized to desmethyldiazepam, an active metabolite of DIAZEPAM.

Clorexolone. Diuretic essentially similar to BENDROFLUAZIDE.

Clorprenaline. Bronchodilator similar to EPHEDRINE.

Clotrimazole. Antifungal agent used topically for skin infections with *Candida.*

Cloxacillin. Penicillinase-resistant PENICILLIN with actions and adverse effects similar to BENZYLPENICILLIN. Use restricted to treatment of penicillinase-producing *Staphylococcus aureus* infections.

Clozapine. Antipsychotic/tranquillizer, used in treatment-resistant schizophrenia. Actions and adverse effects similar to CHLORPROMAZINE but with fewer dopamine antagonist effects and reduced tendency to involuntary movements. Has been associated with bone marrow depression and is used only if haematological monitoring is arranged.

Coal tar. Keratolytic used in topical preparations for eczema and psoriasis.

Coagulation Factor VIIa. Used in haemophilia. Acts to normalise the FACTOR VIII deficiency by bypassing its action rather than by replacement. Adverse reactions include skin irritation, fever, sweating and malaise. May also cause angina, cardiac arrhythmia and hypotension.

Co-amilofruse. Contains AMILORIDE and FRUSEMIDE in a fixed ratio.

Co-amilozide. Contains AMILORIDE and HYDROCHLOROTHIAZIDE in a fixed ratio.

Co-amoxiclav. Contains AMOXYCILLIN and CLAVULANIC ACID in a fixed ratio. May cause liver injury.

Co-beneldopa. Contains BENSERAZIDE and LEVODOPA in a fixed ratio.

Cobalt edetate. *See* DICOBALT EDETATE.

Cobalt tetracemate. *See* DICOBALTEDETATE.

Cocaine (c). Local anaesthetic and sympathomimetic amine. Stabilizes nerve cell membranes to prevent impulse transmission. Little used except topically in eye or respiratory passages. Frequent use may cause corneal ulceration. Stimulates CNS with euphoria and consequent risk of addiction. Chronic misuse leads to delusions, hallucinations, and paranoia.

Co-careldopa. Contains CARBIDOPA and LEVODOPA in a fixed ratio.

Co-codamol. Contains CODEINE and PARACETAMOL in a fixed ratio.

Co-codaprin. Contains CODEINE and ACETYLSALICYLIC ACID in a fixed ratio.

Co-danthramer. Contains DANTHRON and POLOXAMER in a fixed ratio.

Co-danthrusate. Contains DANTHRON and DIOCTYL SODIUM SULPHOSUCCINATE in a fixed ratio.

Codeine. Weak narcotic analgesic. Used for somatic (deep) pain often combined with ACETYLSALICYLIC ACID or PARACETAMOL. Also causes constipation and suppresses the cough reflex. May therefore be used as an anti-diarrhoeal and in cough mixtures. Addiction unusual. Coma with respiratory depression in overdosage. NALOXONE is antidote.

Co-dergocrine. *See* DIHYDROERGOTOXINE.

Cod-liver oil. Oil obtained from fresh cod liver. Used as a source of VITAMINS A and D.

Co-dydramol. Contains DIHYDROCODEINE and PARACETAMOL in a fixed ratio.

Co-fluampicil. Contains FLUCLOXACILLIN and AMPICILLIN in a fixed ratio.

Co-flumactone. Contains HYDROFLUMETHIAZIDE and SPIRONOLACTONE in a fixed ratio.

Colaspase. *See* L-ASPARAGINASE.

Colchicine. Used for relief of pain in acute gout. Adverse effects include nausea, vomiting, colicky pain, and diarrhoea.

Colecalciferol. rINN for CHOLECALCIFEROL.

Colestipol. Ion exchange resin which lowers plasma cholesterol levels through binding with bile acids in the intestinal lumen. Used as an adjunct to diet in treatment of high cholesterol levels. May cause constipation. Must be taken mixed with water or may cause oesophageal damage.

Colestyramine. rINN for CHOLESTYRAMINE.

Colfosceril. A synthetic surfactant used to treat lung damage (Respiratory Distress Syndrome) in preterm infants.

Colistimethate. rINN for COLISTIN.

Colistin. Antibiotic: *see* POLYMYXIN B.

Collagen. Purified bovine collagen injection used as a bulking injection in the periurethral area to reduce stress incontinence at the bladder neck. The additional bulk reduces the urethral luminal space allowing effective contraction of the urethral muscle. Adverse effects include urinary infections, urinary retention and discomfort or bleeding at the site of the injections.

Compound gentian infusion. Bitter extract from the dried root of *Gentiana lutea*. Used to stimulate gastric acid secretion and thus to stimulate appetite.

Co-phenotrope. Contains DIPHENOXYLATE and ATROPINE SULPHATE in a fixed ratio.

Copper acetate. Used topically for its astringent properties.

Copper sulphate. Used as an emetic, together with iron in treatment of anaemia, and as astringent in topical preparations. Large doses may cause copper poisoning. Syrup of IPECACUANHA is generally considered a safer emetic.

Co-prenozide. Contains OXPRENOLOL and CYCLOPENTHIAZIDE in a fixed ratio.

Co-proxamol. Contains DEXTROPROPOXYPHENE and PARACETAMOL in a fixed ratio.

Corticosteroids. General term to include natural and synthetic steroids, with actions similar to HYDROCORTISONE, which is produced in the adrenal cortex. They possess anti-inflammatory and salt-retaining properties. Adverse effects include oedema, hypertension, diabetes, bone thinning with fractures, muscle wasting, infections, and psychosis.

Corticotrophin. Pituitary hormone that controls functions of adrenal cortex.

Corticotropin. rINN for CORTICOTROPHIN.

Cortisone. Naturally occurring adrenal (glucocorticoid) steroid hormone. Has effects upon fat, protein and carbohydrate metabolism, and possesses marked anti-inflammatory activity. Used for replacement therapy in adrenal insufficiency, anti-inflammatory activity in a wide range of conditions, and immunosuppression after organ transplantation or in certain leukaemias. Adverse effects include retention of salt and water, fulminating infections, osteoporosis, peptic ulceration, muscle wasting, hypertension, diabetes mellitus, weight gain, moon face, cataracts, and psychiatric disturbance. On withdrawal of large doses after long periods of treatment there may be failure of the natural adrenal hormone secretion.

Co-simalcite. Contains ACTIVATED DIMETHICONE and HYDROTALCITE in a fixed ratio.

Co-tenidone. Contains ATENOLOL and CHLORTHALIDONE in a fixed ratio.

Co-trimazine. Antibacterial. Combination of SULPHADIAZINE and TRIMETHOPRIM. Actions and adverse effects similar to CO-TRIMOXAZOLE but SULPHADIAZINE is metabolized less than SULPHAMETHOXAZOLE resulting in higher drug concentrations in kidneys and urine. Used for urinary tract infections.

Co-trimoxazole. Antimicrobial. Combination of SULPHAMETHOXAZOLE and TRIMETHOPRIM. Broad antibacterial spectrum, active against typhoid fever. Adverse effects include rashes and blood dyscrasias.

Cresol. Antiseptic. Used as disinfectant or preservative and also as an inhalant for relief of congestion in bronchitis, asthma, and the common cold. If ingested in concentrated solutions, there may be local corrosion, depression of the CNS, and damage to the liver and kidneys.

Crotamiton. Topical treatment for scabies.

Cyanocobalamin. Largely replaced by HYDROXOCOBALAMIN.

Cyclizine. Antihistamine, with actions similar to PROMETHAZINE. Main use as antiemetic.

Cyclobarbitone (c). Barbiturate hypnotic, with actions, uses, and adverse effects similar to AMYLOBARBITONE.

Cyclofenil. Sex hormone used in treatment of infertility due to failure of ovulation. Contraindications and adverse effects similar to CLOMIPHENE.

Cyclopenthiazide. Thiazide diuretic similar to BENDROFLUAZIDE.

Cyclopentolate. Anticholinergic, with actions and adverse effects similar to ATROPINE SULPHATE but with more rapid onset and shorter duration. Used as eye drops to dilate the pupil and to assist optical refraction.

Cyclophosphamide. Cytotoxic used in wide variety of neoplastic diseases. Activated by metabolism in the liver and excreted mainly in the urine. Adverse effects include baldness, cystitis, and renal and bone marrow toxicity.

Cyclopropane. Potent inhalational anaesthetic. Used to induce anaesthesia in paediatric and obstetric practice.

Cycloserine. Antibiotic used in tuberculosis and in *Escherichia coli* and *Proteus* infections. Adverse effects include ataxia, drowsiness, and convulsions.

Cyclosporin. Potent immunosuppressant antibiotic used to prevent rejection after organ and tissue transplantation. Also used to treat severe rheumatoid arthritis, severe psoriasis unresponsive to conventional treatment and severe atopic dermatitis when other treatments fail. Adverse effects include impairment of liver and renal function.

Cycrimine. Parasympatholytic used in treatment of parkinsonism. Similar actions, etc. to BENZHEXOL.

Cyproheptadine. Antihistamine similar to PROMETHAZINE. Stimulates appetite.

Cyproterone. Hormone with antiandrogenic and some progestogenic activity used in the treatment of prostatic carcinoma. Has also been used in sexual disorders in the male, acne, and hirsutism. May cause gynaecomastia, galactorrhoea, sedation, mood changes, altered hair pattern, skin rashes, weight gain, headache, anaemia, liver toxicity and fluctuations in blood pressure. Also avoided in liver disease, thromboembolic disorders, diabetes, and immature youths.

Cysteamine. Formerly used intravenously as an antidote for PARACETAMOL where it acts as a facilitator of glutathione synthesis and thus replenishes the stores necessary to detoxify PARACETAMOL metabolites. Currently used orally in the treatment of the rare inherited metabolic disorder cystinosis where it binds with the amino-acid cystine and reduces its accumulation. May cause troublesome nausea and vomiting.

Cysteine. Amino acid containing sulphur.

Cytarabine (Cytosine arabinoside). Antiviral agent used systemically for herpes encephalitis. Cytotoxic, used in treatment of leukaemia and Hodgkin's disease. Adverse effects include bone marrow depression.

Cytosine arabinoside. *See* CYTARABINE.

D

Dacarbazine. Cytotoxic. May cause bone marrow suppression.

Dactinomycin. *See* ACTINOMYCIN D.

Dakin's solution. Contains calcium hypochlorite, SODIUM BICARBONATE, BORIC ACID. Used as wound disinfectant.

Danaparoid sodium. Low molecular weight heparinoid used for prevention of deep vein thrombosis. Actions, adverse effects and precautions similar to HEPARIN.

Danazol. Used in endocrine disturbances where pituitary control of gonad hormone production is required.

Danthron. Purgative, with actions etc. similar to CASCARA. Use limited to elderly or terminally ill patients because of some incidence of tumour formation in animals at high doses.

Dantrolene. Used in control of skeletal muscle spasticity. Adverse effects include sedation, weakness, and diarrhoea.

Dantron. rINN for DANTHRON.

Dapsone. Sulphone drug used in treatment of leprosy and dermatitis herpetiformis. Adverse effects include allergic dermatitis, nausea, vomiting, tachycardia, haemolytic anaemia, and liver damage.

Daunomycin. *See* DAUNORUBICIN.

Daunorubicin (Rubidomycin, Daunomycin). Cytotoxic antibiotic used in neoplastic disease. Adverse effects include cardiotoxicity and bone marrow depression.

Debrisoquine. Adrenergic neurone blocking drug used in hypertension. Adverse effects as for GUANETHIDINE.

Deglycyrrhizinised liquorice. Mild anti-inflammatory agent. Used in treatment of peptic ulcer. Adverse effects include oedema and hypertension.

Dehydrocholic acid. Used to stimulate secretion of bile flow without increasing its content of bile solids (e.g., after surgery of biliary tract).

Demecarium. Anticholinesterase used by instillation into eye in glaucoma. Actions those of ACETYLCHOLINE.

Demeclocycline. *See* DEMETHYLCHLORTETRACYCLINE.

Demethylchlortetracycline. Bacteriostatic antibiotic with actions, adverse effects, and interactions similar to TETRACYCLINE.

Deoxyribonuclease. Animal pancreatic enzyme used to resolve clots and exudates associated with trauma and inflammation.

Deptropine. Antihistamine similar to PROMETHAZINE.

Dequalinium. Topical antibacterial/antifungal used in oral infections.

Deserpidine. *See* RESERPINE.

Desferrioxamine. Binds with iron. Used orally and parenterally in treatment of acute iron poisoning and in conditions associated with excessive iron storage in tissues, where it increases urinary iron excretion. Adverse effects include allergic reactions.

Desipramine. Antidepressant. Active metabolite of IMIPRAMINE, whose actions and adverse effects it shares.

Desmopressin. Synthetic form of VASOPRESSIN for use nasally in diabetes insipidus and nocturnal enuresis. Acts as an analogue of VASOPRESSIN (antidiuretic hormone), thus counteracts the high volumes of urine produced in both conditions. Destroyed by gastric acid, but is well absorbed via the nasal mucosa.

Desogestrel. Sex hormone, with actions and adverse effects similar to PROGESTERONE. Used for oral contraception in combination with an oestrogenic hormone.

Desonide. Topical corticosteroid for psoriasis and eczema.

Desoximetasone. rINN for DESOXYMETHASONE.

Desoxymethasone. CORTICOSTEROID for topical skin use. Actions and adverse effects similar to DEXAMETHASONE.

Dexamethasone. Potent synthetic CORTICOSTEROID with actions, etc. similar to CORTISONE. Anti-inflammatory activity is much increased in potency, with no increase in salt and water-retaining activity.

Dexamfetamine. rINN for DEXAMPHETAMINE.

Dexamphetamine (c). *See* AMPHETAMINE.

Dexfenfluramine. Dextro-isomer of FENFLURAMINE. More active serotonin agonist than the laevo-isomer and thus has greater effect in reducing obesity than the d-l mixture FENFLURAMINE. Claimed to have a greater effect in reducing obesity but with lower incidence of adverse effects. Has been associated with cardiac valve anomalies in some asymptomatic patients.

Dextranomer. Spherical beads of dextran for surface application to skin wounds. Takes up fluid exudate by capillary action and aids removal of bacteria and tissue debris, thus improving wound healing.

Dextrans. Polysaccharides used intravenously instead of blood or plasma to maintain blood volume and assist capillary flow. Used also as a lubricant in drops for dry eyes. Adverse effects include allergic reactions.

Dextromethorphan. Cough suppressant. Adverse effects include slight psychic dependence and abuse.

Dextromoramide (c). Narcotic analgesic essentially similar to MORPHINE but more reliable when taken by mouth. Useful in the management of severe chronic pain in terminal disease.

Dextropropoxyphene. Weak narcotic analgesic with potency less than CODEINE. Used in moderate pain, commonly with PARACETAMOL when the latter drug is not fully effective. In normal doses, causes less nausea, vomiting, and constipation than codeine. Coma with depressed respiration in overdosage. NALOXONE is antagonist.

Dextrose. Carbohydrate used orally or intravenously as a source of calories in cases of undernutrition. Readily absorbed from the gastro-intestinal tract. Metabolized by energy-producing pathways or stored in the liver as glycogen. Concentrated solutions by mouth may cause nausea and vomiting, intravenously may cause thrombophlebitis.

Diamorphine (Heroin) (c). Narcotic analgesic similar to MORPHINE. Less likely to cause nausea, vomiting, constipation, and hypotension, but greater euphoriant action makes it more addicting and liable to greater abuse.

Diamthazole. Topical antifungal agent. Adverse effects include convulsions if absorbed.

Diazepam (m). Benzodiazepine minor tranquillizer (anxiolytic)/hypnotic with anticonvulsant properties. Acts centrally on the limbic system. Used in treatment of anxiety and as a hypnotic. Useful also in reduction of muscle tone in spasticity and as an anticonvulsant given intravenously for status epilepticus. May cause ataxia, nystagmus and sedation. May impair psychomotor performance. Caution required if driving or operating machinery. Coma in overdosage but little respiratory depression. No antidote. Supportive treatment is adequate. May cause dependence, even in therapeutic doses.

Diazoxide. Used to reduce blood pressure in severe hypertension and to increase blood sugar level in hypoglycaemia. Adverse effects include excessive hair growth, nausea, vomiting, oedema, diabetes, and hypotension.

Dibromopropamidine. Topical antibacterial/antifungal.

Dichloralphenazone. Hypnotic. Combination of CHLORAL HYDRATE and PHENAZONE. Converted back to parent compounds by the liver. Used for insomnia especially in children and the elderly. Relatively 'safe'. Addiction is rare, but rashes and blood disorders may be caused by PHENAZONE. Withdrawn.

Dichlorofluoromethane. *See* CHLOROFLUOROMETHANE.

Dichlorophen. Used in treatment of tapeworms. Adverse effects include nausea, vomiting, and bowel colic.

Dichlorphenamide. Used in treatment of respiratory failure from chronic bronchitis and in glaucoma. Adverse effects include electrolyte imbalance.

Diclofenac. Non-steroid anti-inflammatory/analgesic/antipyretic used in treatment of rheumatoid arthritis and osteoarthritis. Adverse effects include gastro-intestinal upsets, headache, and dizziness.

Dicobalt edetate (Cobalt edetate, Cobalt tetracemate). Antidote for cyanide poisoning. Binds with cyanide and prevents its effects upon cell metabolism.

Dicophane. Insecticide used as dusting powder and lotion for fleas and lice. Very toxic if absorbed.

Dicoumarol. Anticoagulant, with actions, interactions, and adverse effects similar to WARFARIN.

Dicyclomine. Parasympatholytic used in spasm of gastro-intestinal and urinary tracts and to reduce gastric acid in peptic ulceration. Actions, etc. similar to ATROPINE but weaker.

Dicycloverine. rINN for DICYCLOMINE.

Didanosine. Antiviral drug which prevents replication of the human immunodeficiency virus (HIV) involved in AIDS. Adverse reactions include peripheral neuropathy, pancreatitis, gastro-intestinal upset. More rarely, blood dycrasias, liver failure and changes to the optic nerve or retina.

Dienestrol. rINN for DIENOESTROL.

Dienoestrol. Synthetic female sex hormone used for menopausal symptoms and for suppressing lactation. Adverse effects include nausea, vaginal bleeding, and oedema.

Diethylamine salicylate. Rubefacient with actions similar to SALICYLIC ACID.

Diethylcarbamazine. Used in filariasis. Adverse effects include anorexia, nausea, vomiting and encephalopathy. Allergic reactions may accompany release of foreign proteins on death of the worms.

Diethylpropion (c). Anorectic/sympathomimetic amine. Actions those of AMPHETAMINE but less central stimulation and abuse potential.

Diethylstilbestrol. rINN for STILBOESTROL.

Diflucortolone. CORTICOSTEROID for topical use in inflammatory skin conditions. Actions and adverse effects similar to CORTISONE.

Diflunisal. Analgesic related to ACETYLSALICYLIC ACID, but with longer duration of action and no effects on blood platelet function. May cause gastro-intestinal symptoms including ulceration and bleeding, although less common than with ACETYLSALICYLIC ACID. Should not be used if there is a history of hypersensitivity to ACETYLSALICYLIC ACID.

Digitalis. Crude foxglove extract, with same actions, etc. as DIGOXIN but content of active drug is less reliable.

Digitoxin. Foxglove derivative, with similar actions, etc. to DIGOXIN.

Digoxin. Foxglove derivative. Increases force of contraction of heart and slows heart rate, thus making cardiac function more efficient. Used in heart failure and certain abnormal heart rhythms. Influenced by serum potassium levels and by kidney function. In therapeutic overdose, causes vomiting, abdominal pain, diarrhoea, impaired colour vision, slow heart rate, and abnormal heart rhythms.

Digoxin-specific antibody. Fragment (F(ab)) of sheep antibody specific for DIGOXIN and related cardiac drugs. Used to reverse digoxin toxicity by the antibody/antigen reaction which removes the drug and prevents its effects at tissue sites. Given intravenously in a dose determined by the digoxin dose taken. The antibody/antigen complexes are excreted in the urine.

Dihydrocodeine. Mild narcotic analgesic similar to CODEINE, but more potent in relief of pain and more likely to cause constipation. (c) if given by injection.

Dihydroergocornine. *See* DIHYDROERGOTOXINE.

Dihydroergocristine. *See* DIHYDROERGOTOXINE.

Dihydroergokryptine. *See* DIHYDROERGOTOXINE.

Dihydroergotamine. For migraine. Drops, tablets, or intramuscular injection. Used both for prevention and for symptomatic treatment. Has vasoconstrictor effects similar to ERGOTAMINE but milder and with much reduced tendency to hypertension or effects on the uterus. No evidence of ergotism on prolonged or excessive use.

Dihydroergotoxine. Mixture of DIHYDROERGOCORNINE, DIHYDROERGOCRISTINE, and DIHYDROERGOKRYPTINE – ergot derivatives that are alpha-adrenoceptor blockers and vasodilators – used in peripheral and cerebral vascular disease. Adverse effects include nausea and nasal stuffiness.

Dihydrotachysterol. Closely related to VITAMIN D and has similar actions. Used in treatment of rickets and osteomalacia resistant to VITAMIN D. Also used in treatment of osteodystrophy due to chronic renal failure and in hypoparathyroidism. Contraindicated in hypercalcaemia, where it may cause ectopic calcification and renal failure.

Di-iodohydroxyquinoline. Used orally for amoebiasis and topically as skin antiseptic.

Diloxanide. Used in the treatment of intestinal amoebiasis, usually in combination with other drugs. Adverse effects include flatulence, vomiting, pruritus.

Diltiazem. For treatment and prevention of angina and mild to moderate hypertension. Blocks calcium entry into heart muscle and prevents the heart from 'overworking' during exercise. Contraindicated in patients with slow heart rates and poor conduction of cardiac impulse. Adverse effects may include heart block, ankle swelling, nausea, rash, and headache.

Dimenhydrinate. Antihistamine/antiemetic with actions similar to PROMETHAZINE.

Dimercaprol. Binds to heavy metals. Used parenterally in treatment of heavy metal poisoning to increase urinary metal excretion. Adverse effects include nausea, vomiting, and hypertension.

Dimethicone. Used in protective creams and in antacid preparations. Consists of finely divided silicone polymers. In the gut reduces surface tension of small gas bubbles. This allows them to coalesce into larger pockets of gas which are more easily expelled.

Dimethisoquin. Topical local anaesthetic used in lotions and ointments. Adverse effects include allergy and eye irritation.

Dimethyl sulfoxide. rINN for DIMETHYL SULPHOXIDE.

Dimethyl sulphoxide. Used as a solvent in pharmaceutical manufacture. Used alone to reduce inflammation, for example, in the bladder.

Dimeticone. rINN for DIMETHICONE.

Dinoprost (Prostaglandin $F_2\alpha$). Used for induction of abortion.

Dinoprostone (Prostaglandin E_2). Used for induction of abortion and of labour. Prostaglandins are produced in the ovary and uterus with rising concentrations in blood and amniotic fluid at term and during labour. A sustained release pessary formulation may be used to produce gradual effects. Adverse effects include protracted painful uterine contractions. Contraindicated if there has been previous uterine surgery or complications of pregnancy.

Dioctyl sodium sulphosuccinate. Purgative. Lowers surface tension of faecal mass allowing water to penetrate and soften faecal matter. Should not be given together with mineral oil laxatives (e.g., LIQUID PARAFFIN) as this drug may enhance absorption of the oil.

Diphenhydramine. Antihistamine drug, with actions similar to PROMETHAZINE.

Diphenoxylate. Reduces gut motility. Used in control of diarrhoea. Related to MORPHINE; adverse effects include drowsiness, euphoria, respiratory depression, coma, and dependence.

Diphenylpyraline. Antihistamine similar to PROMETHAZINE.

Dipipanone (c). Narcotic analgesic essentially similar to METHADONE.

Dipivefrine. Pro-drug, metabolized to ADRENALINE after absorption. Used as eye drops for chronic open-angle glaucoma where the pro-drug passes through the cornea more readily than adrenaline. May cause transitory stinging of the eyes.

Diprophylline. Bronchodilator, with actions similar to AMINOPHYLLINE.

Dipyridamole. Used in treatment of angina. Reduces platelet stickiness. Adverse effects include flushing, headache, and hypotension.

Disopyramide. Used in abnormal heart rhythms. Adverse effects include dry mouth, blurred vision, and urinary hesitancy.

Distigmine. Anticholinesterase: *see* NEOSTIGMINE.

Disulfiram. Blocks alcohol metabolism at stage of acetaldehyde. Produces nausea, vomiting, severe headache, chest pain, dyspnoea, hypotension, and collapse if taken before alcohol. Used in treatment of alcoholism. Other adverse effects include impotence, neuropathy, and interference with anticoagulant activity of WARFARIN.

Dithranol. Used topically in psoriasis and other chronic skin conditions where it is thought to act by reducing the rate of skin cell formation. Adverse effects include staining of clothes and severe irritation to the eyes and skin.

Dobutamine. Synthetic beta-adrenoceptor agonist chemically similar to ISOPRENALINE. Stimulates cardiac beta-adrenoceptors directly causing an increase in cardiac output with less increase in cardiac rate than with isoprenaline. Used as infusion in treatment of shock. Unlike DOPAMINE does not cause constriction of peripheral blood vessels and rise in blood pressure but lacks the favourable effect of the latter on renal blood flow. May cause cardiac arrhythmias, but less frequently than with ISOPRENALINE.

Docetaxel. Cytotoxic. A semi-synthetic derivative of a natural substance (taxoid) found in the Pacific yew tree. Most active against rapidly growing tumours, it is used in locally advanced or metastatic breast cancer. Adverse effects include bone marrow suppression, bleeding, rashes and a wide range of systemic effects.

Docusate sodium. Laxative. Promotes water penetration into faeces with softening and increased rate of transit along large bowel.

Domiphen. Topical disinfectant used in skin and mouth preparations.

Domperidone. Antiemetic, with dopamine antagonist actions similar to METOCLOPRAMIDE. Used to control nausea and vomiting due to cancer chemotherapy. Adverse effects include drowsiness, involuntary movements, and cardiac dysrhythmias.

Donepezil. Central acetylcholinesterase inhibitor used to provide symptomatic relief in mild cases of Alzheimer's disease. Acts by inhibiting breakdown of acetylcholine in the brain and thus helping to compensate for the central deficiency that is a feature of the disease. May cause nausea, vomiting, dizziness, insomnia, fatigue and muscle cramps. Peripheral anticholinesterase effects are low but caution is needed in cases with known bladder outflow obstruction, gastric ulceration, and asthma.

Dopamine. Naturally occurring precursor of NORADRENALINE that possesses sympathomimetic properties in its own right. Used intravenously in treatment of shock where it increases cardiac output with less risk of arrhythmias than ISOPRENALINE. Unlike DOBUTAMINE or ISOPRENALINE has a vasodilator action on blood vessels to kidneys and may help to improve kidney function. Larger doses may cause peripheral vasoconstriction with a rise in pressure (*see* DOBUTAMINE).

Dopexamine. Beta-adrenoreceptor agonist which increases cardiac output and increases blood flow to peripheral blood vessels and blood vessels in the kidney. Unlike DOPAMINE it does not produce vasoconstriction at high doses. May produce nausea, vomiting and tachycardia at high doses.

Dornase alfa. Synthetic (recombinant) enzyme that breaks down the DNA content of purulent sputum. Used by inhalation in cystic fibrosis to assist in clearing sputum from the lungs. Adverse effects include pharyngitis/laryngitis and skin rash.

Dorzolamide. Carbonic anhydrase enzyme inhibitor with actions similar to ACETAZOLAMIDE but with better ocular penetration when used topically. Used as eye drops for treatment of open-angle glaucoma, alone or in conjunction with a topical beta-adrenoceptor blocking drug. Adverse effects include a bitter taste, conjunctivitis, blurred vision and headache.

Dosulepin. rINN for DOTHIEPIN.

Dothiepin. Tricyclic antidepressant, with actions, uses, etc. similar to IMIPRAMINE. Also has mild tranquillizing action, which may be useful in agitated depression. May cause extrapyramidal adverse effects.

Doxapram. CNS stimulant used to stimulate respiration. Adverse effects include convulsions and abnormal heart rhythms.

Doxazosin. Long-acting antihypertensive with alpha-adrenoceptor blocking effects. May also be used to reduce symptoms of urinary obstruction caused by benign prostatic hypertrophy. Adverse effects include dizziness, vertigo, headache, fatigue, asthenia, oedema and rarely, incontinence. Similar in action to PRAZOSIN.

Doxepin. Tricyclic antidepressant, with actions, uses, etc. similar to IMIPRAMINE. Also has mild tranquillizing effect which may relieve anxiety associated with depression.

Doxorubicin. Cytotoxic antibiotic used in neoplastic disease. Adverse effects include bone marrow depression, cardiotoxicity, and gastro-intestinal disturbances.

Doxycycline. Bacteriostatic antibiotic, with actions, adverse effects, and interactions similar to TETRACYCLINE. Unlike other tetracyclines, is not excreted by kidneys. Therefore used where renal impairment is a complication. The capsule formulation is apt to stick to the oesophageal mucosa where it dissolves and causes mucosal damage due to high acidity. A soluble formulation is available.

Doxylamine. Antihistamine similar to PROMETHAZINE.

Droperidol. Butyrophenone tranquillizer, with actions and adverse effects similar to HALOPERIDOL. Used in combination with analgesics such as PHENOPERIDINE to maintain the patient in a state of neurolept-analgesia – calm and indifferent while conscious and able to cooperate with the surgeon.

Drostanolone. Anabolic steroid given by intramuscular injection. Adverse effects as for TESTOSTERONE.

D-Xylose. Sugar similar to glucose. Readily absorbed from the normal small intestine but has low rate of metabolism with consequent excretion of approximately 30 per cent unchanged in the urine. Used as a test for intestinal malabsorption since lower absorption results in lower levels in the urine. May cause diarrhoea, nausea, and abdominal discomfort.

Dydrogesterone. Actions similar to PROGESTERONE, but does not inhibit ovulation and does not have contraceptive effect.

Dyflos. Organophosphorus, long-acting anticholinesterase, with actions, etc. similar to PHYSOSTIGMINE.

E

Econazole. Antifungal agent, with actions, uses, and adverse effects similar to MICONAZOLE.

Ecothiopate. Anticholinesterase similar to DYFLOS.

Edrophonium. Short-acting anticholinesterase, with actions similar to PHYSOSTIGMINE. Used in diagnosis of myasthenia gravis.

Eformoterol. Selective beta-2 adrenoceptor agonist with actions similar to SALBUTAMOL, but of longer duration. Adverse effects include tremor, headache, palpitations, tachycardia, and muscle cramps. Used by inhalation in patients requiring long-term therapy for asthma.

Egg phosphatide. *See* LECITHINS.

Embramine. Antihistamine similar to PROMETHAZINE.

Emetine. Anti-amoebic agent given by subcutaneous injection. Adverse effects include nausea, vomiting, hypotension, and cardiac arrhythmias.

Enalapril. Antihypertensive, with actions, uses, and adverse effects similar to CAPTOPRIL.

Enflurane. Inhalation anaesthetic similar to HALOTHANE.

Enoxaparin. A low molecular weight HEPARIN prepared by fractionating naturally occurring heparin. Has increased effect against thrombus (clot) formation but with less tendency to haemorrhagic adverse effects. *See* HEPARIN.

Enoximone. Increases cardiac output by increasing stroke volume and reducing venous pressure without significant increase in heart rate. Used intravenously in heart failure refractory to other drugs. May cause hypotension, headache and insomnia. Gastro-intestinal symptoms, fever and urinary retention may also occur.

Ephedrine (m). Sympathomimetic amine with alpha- and beta-adrenoceptor effects. Bronchodilator used in bronchial asthma. Also as mydriatic and nasal decongestant. Adverse effects include tachycardia, anxiety, and insomnia.

Epinephrine. rINN for ADRENALINE.

Epirubicin. Cytotoxic antibiotic with uses, actions, and adverse effects similar to DOXORUBICIN.

Epoetin alfa. A synthetic preparation of human erythropoietin hormone, normally produced by the kidneys, which increases red blood cell production. Used to treat anaemia in patients with chronic renal failure on dialysis, where the kidney is no longer able to produce sufficient hormone, and anaemia caused by chemotherapy with platinum-containing compounds. Adverse effects include raised blood pressure, thrombosis at injection sites, influenza-like symptoms, convulsions, and skin reactions.

Epoetin beta. Hormone preparation similar to EPOETIN ALFA.

Epoprostenol (Prostacyclin, PGI_2). Endogenously produced prostaglandin with potent vasodilator properties. Administered intravenously. Inhibits platelet aggregation.

Preserves platelet function during cardiac bypass procedures and charcoal haemoperfusion. May be used as anticoagulant, alternative to heparin in renal dialysis. Adverse effects include headache, flushing, hypotension.

Epsom salts. *See* MAGNESIUM SULPHATE.

Ergocalciferol. Form of VITAMIN D obtained from fungi and yeasts.

Ergometrine. Derivative of ergot – a fungus which grows on rye. Causes contraction of uterine muscle. Used in obstetrics after delivery of the baby to prevent or reduce maternal haemorrhage. Adverse effects as for ERGOTAMINE.

Ergotamine. Ergot derivative similar to ERGOMETRINE but with vasoconstricting and alpha-adrenoceptor blocking activity. Used in treatment of migraine by oral, intramuscular, sublingual, aerosol, or suppository routes. Adverse effects include nausea, vomiting, headache, convulsions, and cold extremities. Rarely, may cause myocardial infarct in patients with no known history of coronary heart disease.

Erythromycin. Bactericidal antibiotic, with spectrum of activity similar to BENZYLPENICILLIN, plus some strains of *Haemophilus influenzae* and mycoplasmas. Adverse effects include diarrhoea and liver damage with jaundice. Used systemically for a wide range of infections, especially in penicillin-sensitive individuals. Also used topically for treatment of mild to moderate acne.

Eserine. *See* PHYSOSTIGMINE.

Essential oils. Volatile, odorous mixtures of plant origin with a mild irritant effect on skin and mucous membranes. Used as carminatives for the gastro-intestinal tract (induce feelings of warmth and salivation), or as counter-irritants on the skin (cause warmth and smarting). Also widely used as flavours and in 'traditional' medicines.

Estradiol. rINN for OESTRADIOL.

Estramustine phosphate. Cytotoxic drug used in neoplastic disease. Adverse effects include lower abdominal burning sensation and bone marrow depression.

Estriol. rINN for OESTRIOL.

Estrone. rINN for OESTRONE.

Etacrynic acid. rINN for ETHACRYNIC ACID.

Etamsylate. rINN for ETHAMSYLATE.

Ethacrynic acid. Potent diuretic. Action and uses similar to FRUSEMIDE. Adverse effects similar to BENDROFLUAZIDE. May also cause transient deafness.

Ethambutol. Anti-tuberculous drug. Well tolerated but high doses toxic to optic nerve, producing central or periaxial retrobulbar neuritis.

Ethamivan. Respiratory stimulant essentially similar to NIKETHAMIDE. May be used in respiratory depression of the newborn.

Ethamsylate. Haemostatic agent used to control surgical and menstrual blood loss.

Ethanolamine. Sclerosing agent used in t he injection treatment of varicose veins. Contraindicated if there is thrombophlebitis. May cause hypersensitivity allergic reactions.

Ethinylestradiol. rINN for ETHINYLOESTRADIOL.

Ethinyloestradiol. Synthetic female sex hormone with similar actions and adverse effects to DIENOESTROL. Combined with progestational drug in some oral contraceptives and in treatment of acne and hirsutism.

Ethionamide. Anti-tuberculous agent. High incidence of adverse effects, mainly on gastro-intestinal tract.

Ethisterone. Similar actions and adverse effects to PROGESTERONE.

Ethoheptazine. Analgesic for mild to moderate pain. Adverse effects include nausea and drowsiness.

Ethomoxane. Alpha-adrenoceptor blocking drug similar to PHENTOLAMINE.

Ethopropazine. Parasympatholytic used in treatment of parkinsonism. Less effective than BENZHEXOL and causes more frequent side effects.

Ethosalmide. Analgesic, with similar actions and adverse effects to SALICYLAMIDE.

Ethosuximide. Anticonvulsant. Suppresses epileptic discharges in the brain. Used in treatment of petit mal (absence seizures) but not for major epilepsy. May cause nausea and vomiting, drowsiness or excitation, photophobia, and Parkinson-like symptoms. Coma with respiratory depression in overdosage. No antidote. Supportive treatment only.

Ethotoin. Anticonvulsant essentially similar to PHENYTOIN but less toxic and less effective.

Ethyl biscoumacetate. Anticoagulant drug, with actions similar to WARFARIN.

Ethylene diamine. Pharmaceuticalaid used in manufacture of AMINOPHYLLINE, and of some creams for topical application. Can produce allergic dermatitis by both topical and systemic administration.

Ethyl nicotinate. Topical vasodilator. *See* NICOTINIC ACID.

Ethyloestrenol. Anabolic steroid. Adverse effects as for TESTOSTERONE.

Ethyl salicylate. Similar to METHYL SALICYLATE.

Ethynodiol. Similar actions and adverse effects to PROGESTERONE. Combined with oestrogenic agent in some oral contraceptives.

Etidronate. A biphosphonate which influences bone structure and strength by increasing bone mass and reducing bone reabsorption. Used to treat osteoporosis and Paget's disease of bone (osteitis deformans). Adverse effects include diarrhoea and nausea.

Etodolac. Non-steroid anti-inflammatory/analgesic, with actions and uses similar to IBUPROFEN. Adverse effects include gastro-intestinal intolerance, but claimed to produce less gastric bleeding than other drugs in this group.

Etomidate. Used by injection for induction of anaesthesia. May cause pain on injection, hypotension and involuntary movements.

Etoposide. Cytotoxic drug used in treatment of malignant disease. Adverse effects include nausea, vomiting, and bone marrow depression.

Etretinate. Synthetic derivative of retinoic acid (VITAMIN A) used in treatment of severe intractable psoriasis and some other serious disorders of skin growth. Adverse effects include teratogenic actions, dryness of mouth and other mucous membranes, exfoliation of the skin, hair loss, and disorders of liver function and blood fats. Acute overdosage produces severe headache, nausea, vomiting and drowsiness, requiring immediate withdrawal of the drug and non-specific supportive treatment. Contraindicated in pregnancy.

Etynodiol. rINN for ETHYNODIOL.

Eucalyptus. Essential oil used internally to relieve catarrh and externally as rubefacient.

Eucatropine. Parasympatholytic mydriatic similar to HOMATROPINE.

F

Factor VIII. Blood clotting factor that is deficient in haemophilia and Von Willebrand's disease. Used intravenously to stop episodes of uncontrollable bleeding.

Factor IX concentrate. HIV-free clotting factor purified and concentrated from human blood plasma. May cause headache, fever, flushing, vomiting and thromboembolic episodes.

Famciclovir. Antiviral agent used orally to treat herpes zoster infections, shingles and genital herpes. It is a prodrug, which is rapidly metabolised to its active metabolite PENCICLOVIR, in the liver. Should only be used with caution in patients with renal impairment. Adverse effects include headache and nausea.

Famotidine. Gastric histamine receptor blocker, with actions and uses similar to CIMETIDINE, but longer duration of action. May cause tiredness, headache, dizziness, constipation, diarrhoea, anorexia, and other minor gastro-intestinal symptoms.

Felbinac. Non-steroid anti-inflammatory/analgesic derived from FENBUFEN, for topical application after soft-tissue injury. It acts locally and has minimal systemic effects. It may cause mild local erythema, dermatitis and pruritus. It is contraindicated in hypersensitivity to ACETYLSALICYLIC ACID.

Felodipine. Calcium antagonist with actions and adverse effects similar to NIFEDIPINE. Used to treat hypertension and angina.

Felypressin. Vasoconstrictor polypeptide used in some local anaesthetic preparations. Less likely than sympathomimetic vasoconstrictors to cause cardiac arrhythmias, and does not interact with antidepressant drugs.

Fenbufen. Non-steroid anti-inflammatory/analgesic, with action and uses similar to IBUPROFEN. Has long duration of action and needs only twice daily dosage. Adverse effects include gastro-intestinal intolerance, skin rashes, dizziness and headaches. Contraindicated in hypersensitivity to ACETYLSALICYLIC ACID.

Fenclofenac. Anti-inflammatory/analgesic, with actions, uses, and adverse effects similar to IBUPROFEN.

Fenfluramine. Anti-obesity, with central anorectic and peripheral metabolic effects. Claimed to be effective in autism. May produce diarrhoea, sedation, and sleep disturbance. Contraindicated in patients taking monoamine oxidase inhibitors. Has been associated with cardiac valve abnormalities in some asymptomatic patients.

Fennel. Essential oil used as carminative.

Fenofibrate. Reduces blood cholesterol and fats in patients with raised blood levels which do not respond to changes in diet. Related to CLOFIBRATE but the precise mode of action is unclear. Fewer adverse effects than CLOFIBRATE but may cause gastro-intestinal disturbances, skin rashes and tiredness.

Fenoprofen. Anti-inflammatory/analgesic, with similar actions and uses to INDOMETHACIN.

Fenoterol. Actions and adverse effects similar to SALBUTAMOL.

Fentanyl (c). Narcotic analgesic, with actions and uses similar to MORPHINE. More potent analgesic and respiratory depressant, but shorter action. May be administered transdermally from patches.

Fenticonazole. Antifungal used topically as pessaries for vulvo-vaginal candiasis. Actions and effectiveness similar to MICONAZOLE and CLOTRIMAZOLE. Used as a single dose or on three consecutive nights. May cause local irritation.

Ferric ammonium citrate. Actions and adverse effects similar to FERROUS SULPHATE.

Ferric chloride. Iron salt included in some 'tonics' or treatments for iron deficiency. Actions and adverse effects similar to FERROUS SULPHATE.

Ferric hydroxide. Iron salt, with actions similar to FERROUS SULPHATE.

Ferrous fumarate. Actions and adverse effects similar to FERROUS SULPHATE.

Ferrous gluconate. Actions and adverse effects similar to FERROUS SULPHATE.

Ferrous glycine sulphate. *See* FERROUS SULPHATE.

Ferrous succinate. Actions and adverse effects similar to FERROUS SULPHATE.

Ferrous sulphate. Used as a source of iron to replenish body iron stores in iron deficiency anaemia. Adverse effects include black faeces, abdominal pain, constipation, and diarrhoea. Liquid formulations can stain teeth black.

Fexofenadine. Non-sedative antihistamine used in treatment of hay fever (seasonal allergic rhinitis). Has actions and adverse effects similar to TERFENADINE and ASTEMIZOLE, but appears to lack cardiac effects.

Filgrastim. Human growth factor which stimulates production of white blood cells within the bone marrow. Made by recombinant DNA technology. Used to enhance white blood cell production in patients whose bone marrow function is depressed by cytotoxic treatment. Adverse effects include muscle pain and painful micturition.

Finasteride. Enzyme inhibitor which blocks the formation of the male sex hormone dihydrotestosterone from testosterone. The former is active in promoting benign growth of the prostate gland in older men, whilst the latter maintains male sexual characteristics. Used in the treatment of benign prostatic hypertrophy. Finasteride reduces the size of the gland without causing feminising side-effects. Should not be used to treat cancer of the prostate, as it may cause impotence and decreased libido.

Flavoxate. Antispasmodic used in bladder disorders. Adverse effects include headache and dry mouth.

Flecainide. Antiarrhythmic, with actions and adverse effects similar to LIGNOCAINE but active by mouth. Used to treat and prevent life-threatening, irregular cardiac rhythms.

Flosequinan. Direct-acting vasodilator with effects upon arterioles and veins. Used in treatment of cardiac failure when it reduces the stress on the heart both from venous inflow and resistance to arterial outflow. Acts by relaxing muscles in the blood vessel walls. May cause headaches, dizziness, palpitations, low blood pressure, joint pains, rashes and photosensitivity. Withdrawn due to evidence of increasing risk of hospitalization and mortality of patients with congestive heart failure.

Fluclorolone. Topical CORTICOSTEROID used in psoriasis and eczema.

Flucloxacillin. Antibiotic. Similar properties to CLOXACILLIN, but better absorbed.

Fluconazole. Antifungal agent used to treat vaginal and oral fungal infections. Adverse effects include nausea, headache and abdominal discomfort.

Flucytosine. Antifungal agent active orally against systemic *Candida* infections. Adverse effects include bone marrow depression.

Fludarabine. Cytotoxic used in treatment of chronic lymphocytic leukaemia where it may achieve complete or partial remission. Adverse effects include bone marrow suppression, fever and infection.

Fludrocortisone. Potent salt-retaining CORTICOSTEROID used in adrenal insufficiency. Adverse effects include oedema, hypertension, and electrolyte imbalance.

Fludroxycortide. rINN for FLURANDRENOLONE.

Flufenamic acid. Anti-inflammatory/analgesic essentially similar to MEFENAMIC ACID.

Flumazenil. Benzodiazepine antagonist which completely or partially reverses the central sedative effects. Used to reverse benzodiazepine effects after short diagnostic and therapeutic procedures. Its use in the reversal of benzodiazepine overdose is not yet established, and it is not licensed for this purpose.

Flumetasone. rINN for FLUMETHASONE.

Flumethasone. Topical CORTICOSTEROID used in psoriasis and eczema.

Flunisolide. Potent synthetic CORTICOSTEROID similar to DEXAMETHASONE. Used by nasal spray for treatment of allergic rhinitis.

Flunitrazepam (c). Benzodiazepine hypnotic/ anxiolytic with actions, uses, and adverse effects similar to NITRAZEPAM. Recommended only for short-term treatment of insomnia.

Fluocinolone. Topical CORTICOSTEROID used in psoriasis and eczema.

Fluocinonide. Topical CORTICOSTEROID used in psoriasis and eczema.

Fluocortolone. Topical CORTICOSTEROID used in psoriasis and eczema.

Fluorescein. Staining agent used for detection of damage to the cornea and as a test of pancreatic function.

Fluorometholone. Potent synthetic CORTICOSTEROID, similar to DEXAMETHASONE.

Fluorouracil. Cytotoxic, used in the treatment of metastatic cancer of the colon, breast cancer and other solid tumours. May be used topically for some skin lesions including genital warts. Adverse effects include bone marrow suppression and central nervous system disturbances.

Fluoxetine. Antidepressant which acts by blocking re-uptake of serotonin into nerve cells. It has a lower incidence of noradrenergic and cholinergic side effects than tricyclic antidepressants (e.g., IMIPRAMINE) and is less likely to cause sedation and cardiac side effects. It also seems to be safer in overdose. May cause nausea, headache, insomnia, dizziness, asthenia, rash, convulsions, hypomania and mania.

Flupenthixol. Tranquillizer, with antidepressant and anxiolytic actions but little sedative effects. Used in depressive and anxiety states associated with inertia and apathy. Adverse effects include restlessness, insomnia, hypotension, and extrapyramidal disturbances. Not recommended for children or excitable patients or in advanced cardiac, renal, or hepatic disease.

Flupentixol. rINN for FLUPENTHIXOL.

Fluphenazine. Phenothiazine tranquillizer similar to CHLORPROMAZINE, but longer-acting. Used in treatment of psychoses, confusion, and agitation. Oral treatment required only once a day. Available as a 'depot' intramuscular injection which is active for 10–28 days. Adverse effects similar to CHLORPROMAZINE but more frequently causes involuntary movements.

Fluprednylidene. Topical CORTICOSTEROID used in psoriasis and eczema.

Flurandrenolone. Topical CORTICOSTEROID used in psoriasis and eczema.

Flurazepam. Benzodiazepine tranquillizer/hypnotic. Used in the treatment of insomnia. Essentially similar to NITRAZEPAM.

Flurbiprofen. Anti-inflammatory/analgesic, with actions, uses, and adverse effects similar to IBUPROFEN. Used in inflammatory joint diseases and as eye drops to prevent trauma-induced pupil constriction during eye surgery.

Fluspirilene. Tranquillizer used in schizophrenia. Adverse effects include involuntary movements and low blood pressure.

Flutamide. Anti-androgen used to block effects of male sex hormones on growth of cancer of the prostate gland. May cause gynaecomastia, breast tenderness, and milk production, also gastro-intestinal disturbances and insomnia.

Fluticasone. Potent synthetic CORTICOSTEROID similar to DEXAMETHASONE.

Fluvastatin. Synthetic enzyme inhibitor which suppresses production of cholesterol in the body. Used to treat high blood cholesterol when reduction of dietary intake alone is not sufficient. Adverse effects include dyspepsia, nausea, abdominal pain and flatulence, myalgia and muscle weakness. May also cause insomnia and abnormal liver function tests.

Fluvoxamine. Antidepressant. Acts by blocking re-uptake of serotonin into nerve cells. Does not have anticholinergic effects and thus is less likely to cause cardiac side effects than tricyclic antidepressants (e.g., IMIPRAMINE). May cause nausea, constipation, weight loss, drowsiness, anxiety and tremor. Should not be used with theophylline or aminophylline because it may affect their metabolism and precipitate toxic effects such as nausea, headache, vomiting, and agitation.

Folic acid. Used in folate-deficient megaloblastic anaemias of pregnancy, malnutrition, and malabsorption states. May precipitate neuropathy in untreated HYDROXOCOBALAMIN deficiency.

Folinic acid. Used as an antidote to antifolate cytotoxic agents and in the treatment of megaloblastic anaemias, other than due to vitamin B_{12} (HYDROXOCOBALAMIN) deficiency.

Formaldehyde. As a solution used topically for treatment of warts.

Formestane. Inhibits enzyme involved in production of oestrogen, leading to prolonged suppression of oestrogen secretion in the ovaries and adrenal glands. Used to treat advanced oestrogen-dependent breast cancer. May cause hot flushes, vaginal bleeding, joint pains, fluid retention and gastro-intestinal disturbance.

Foscarnet. Antiviral drug which inhibits the replication of both human immunodeficiency viruses (HIV) involved in AIDS and the herpes viruses. Adverse effects include impaired renal function, hypocalcaemia, hypoglycaemia, epileptic seizures, decrease in haemoglobin concentration, headache, nausea, vomiting and rash.

Fosfomycin. Bactericidal antibiotic that acts by inhibiting bacterial cell wall synthesis. It has a broad spectrum of activity and rapidly achieves high urinary concentrations after oral administration. It is used for prophylaxis and treatment of urinary tract infections. Adverse effects include rashes and gastro-intestinal disturbances.

Fosinopril. Antihypertensive with similar actions to CAPTOPRIL also used to treat congestive heart failure. Adverse effects include dizziness, cough, gastro-intestinal disturbances, palpitations, chest pain, rash, musculoskeletal pain, fatigue, and taste disturbances.

Framycetin. Antibiotic derivative of NEOMYCIN used topically for skin infections and by mouth for gastro-enteritis and bowel sterilization.

Frangula. Mild purgative, with actions, etc. similar to CASCARA.

Frusemide. Potent diuretic which causes greater reduction in sodium reabsorption by the kidney than occurs with the thiazide diuretics (*see* BENDROFLUAZIDE). Rapid onset of action when given orally or intravenously. Used in emergency treatment of fluid overload, especially pulmonary oedema and in cases resistant to thiazides. May also be used as antihypertensive. Adverse effects similar to BENDROFLUAZIDE.

Fuller's earth. Adsorbent. Used in poisoning due to the weedkiller paraquat, which it binds strongly. Administered orally or directly into stomach via naso-gastric tube. May be given with MAGNESIUM SULPHATE to promote diarrhoea and thus attempt to empty the gut of paraquat.

Furazolidone. Poorly absorbed antibacterial drug used in bacterial diarrhoea and gastro-enteritis. Adverse effects include nausea, vomiting, rashes, haemolysis in predisposed patients, and flushing with alcohol.

Furosemide. rINN for FRUSEMIDE.

Fusafungine. Antibiotic administered by aerosol for infections of upper respiratory tract.

Fusidic acid. Steroid antibiotic used for infections by PENICILLIN-resistant *staphylococci*. Adverse effects include nausea and vomiting.

G

Gabapentin. Anticonvulsant. Structurally similar to the neurotransmitter GABA but mode of action uncertain. Used as an adjunct to other anticonvulsant therapy. Adverse effects include drowsiness, dizziness, headache, tremor, nausea and vomiting.

Gallamine. Skeletal muscle relaxant used during surgical procedures under general anaesthesia. Has action similar to TUBOCURARINE.

Gamma-benzene hexachloride. Applied topically for treatment of lice, scabies, and other infestations. Adverse effects include convulsions if ingested.

Gamolenic acid. Essential fatty acid derived from the evening primrose plant for systemic treatment of atopic eczema. May cause nausea, diarrhoea and headache and cyclical or non-cyclical breast pain. Appears to reduce breast pain by reducing sensitivity to cyclical hormone changes.

Ganciclovir. Antiviral agent for cytomegalovirus infections, such as retinitis and pneumonitis, in immunocompromised patients, including those suffering from AIDS. It prevents the virus from replicating and stops the progression of the infection, but it is not a cure and if the treatment is stopped the virus may begin to replicate again. May cause fever, rashes, depression and impairment of liver and kidney function.

Gefarnate. Used for treatment of peptic ulcer. May cause skin rashes.

Gelatin. Protein used as a nutrient in the preparation of some oral medicines and suppositories, and in a sponge-like form as a haemostatic.

Gemcitabine. Cytotoxic used as palliative treatment for non-small cell lung cancer (the major form of that disease in the UK). Adverse effects include bone marrow suppression, nausea, vomiting, fever and muscle pains.

Gemeprost. Synthetic prostaglandin which acts on the uterus to prepare it for delivery of the foetus. Used as a pessary to prepare the uterus for surgical termination of pregnancy.

Gemfibrozil. Reduces blood lipid concentrations, both triglycerides and cholesterol. Used together with diet in patients with proven hyperlipidaemias. Mechanism of action unclear, but probably reduces lipid synthesis in the liver and enhances clearance. May cause abdominal pain, diarrhoea, nausea, vomiting and flatulence. Skin rashes, headaches, blurred vision, impotence and painful extremities have also been described.

Gentamicin. Bactericidal aminoglycoside antibiotic injection with spectrum similar to NEOMYCIN, but specially active against *Pseudomonas aeruginosa.* Adverse effects include ototoxicity and nephrotoxicity, particularly in renal failure. Potentiates neuromuscular blockade.

Gestodene. Sex hormone, with actions, uses, and adverse effects similar to NORGESTREL. Combined with oestrogenic agent as an oral contraceptive.

Gestrinone. A synthetic steroid for treatment of endometriosis. Has anti-oestrogenic and androgenic activity which reduces the size of the endometrial tissue fragments, and leads to their regression. May cause temporary suppression of normal menstruation. Adverse effects include acne, fluid retention, nervousness, depression, voice changes and increased hair growth.

Gestronol. Hormone, with similar actions to PROGESTERONE.

Glauber's salts. *See* SODIUM SULPHATE.

Glibenclamide. Oral antidiabetic drug, with actions and uses similar to CHLORPROPAMIDE.

Gliclazide. Oral antidiabetic, with actions, uses, and adverse effects similar to CHLORPROPAMIDE. Also reduces adhesiveness of blood platelets and thus may reduce the cardiovascular complications of diabetes.

Glipizide. Oral antidiabetic drug, with actions and uses similar to CHLORPROPAMIDE.

Gliquidone. Oral antidiabetic, with similar action to CHLORPROPAMIDE but rapidly metabolized by the liver and excreted in the faeces to give a short duration of effects similar to TOLBUTAMIDE. Recommended when there is a greater danger of hypoglycaemia (e.g., in the elderly). Adverse effects include gastro-intestinal upsets and skin rashes.

Glucagon. Polypeptide hormone produced by alpha-cells of pancreas. Causes increase in blood sugar, release of several other hormones, and increases force of cardiac contraction. Used in tests of carbohydrate metabolism and in treatment of heart failure. May cause nausea and vomiting but cardiac arrhythmias are said not to occur.

Glucose. Source of carbohydrate nutrition. Administered by mouth or intravenously as a dietary supplement. Also used acutely to reverse hypoglycaemic attacks associated with diabetes melitus.

Glutaraldehyde. As a solution used to treat warts.

Gluten. Constituent of wheat starch responsible for bowel disorders in gluten-sensitive individuals. These conditions respond to treatment with a gluten-free diet.

Glycerin. Carbohydrate used as a sweetening agent in some mixtures and pastilles and as high-calorie source in intravenous feeds. Used topically in skin preparations for water retaining and softening properties. In suppositories or enemas, it promotes bowel peristalsis and evacuation.

Glycerin suppositories. Local lubricant purgative.

Glycerol. *See* GLYCERIN.

Glycerophosphates. Used widely in 'tonic' preparations as a source of phosphorus.

Glyceryl trinitrate. Vasodilator for symptomatic or prophylactic treatment of angina pectoris. Administered as sublingual tablets or oral spray for rapid absorption at onset of symptoms or applied as gel to skin for sustained absorption in prophylaxis. May also be used intravenously to treat cardiac failure, during hypotensive surgery or during cardiac surgery to prevent myocardial infarction. Adverse effects include headache, dizziness, and flushing. Loses potency if not stored away from light and under cool conditions. Applications to skin may cause local allergic reactions.

Glycine. Amino acid used with antacids in gastric hyperacidity, and with aspirin to reduce its gastric irritation.

Glycol salicylate. Rubefacient. Essentially similar to SALICYLIC ACID.

Glycopyrronium. Anticholinergic similar to ATROPINE, used in peptic ulcer, gastric hyperacidity, and to reduce excessive sweating.

Gold salts. Anti-inflammatory agent, apparently specific for rheumatoid arthritis. Mechanism of action unknown. Given by mouth or as a course of intramuscular injections. Toxic reactions are common including stomatitis, dermatitis, nausea, vomiting, and diarrhoea. May cause hepatitis, nephritis, and bone marrow depression. Not given if evidence of pre-existing liver or kidney disease.

Gonadorelin. Hormone produced in the hypothalamus of the brain which stimulates the ovarian hormones luteinizing hormone (LH) and follicle-stimulating hormone (FSH). Used as pulsatile subcutaneous or intravenous injection for treatment of amenorrhoea and infertility due to ovarian hormone deficiency. May cause gastro-intestinal symptoms, skin rashes, and abdominal pain.

Gonadotrophin. Pituitary hormone that stimulates gonadal activity. Used in infertility and delayed puberty.

Goserelin. Hormone, analogue of gonadotrophin-releasing hormone. Used for depot administration in abdominal wall to treat cancer of the prostate gland, endometriosis and breast cancer. Acts by reducing production of male sex hormones. May cause hot flushes, loss of libido, breast development, bruising at injection site and transient increase in bone pain.

Gramicidin. Antibiotic used by local application to skin, wounds, burns, and nose and mouth infections. Toxic if ingested or injected.

Granisetron. Potent antiemetic with actions similar to ONDANSETRON.

Grepafloxacin. Oral broad spectrum antibiotic with actions, uses and adverse effects similar to CIPROFLOXACIN.

Griseofulvin. Antibiotic active against fungal infections of skin and nails when taken orally. May require higher doses in patients on anticonvulsant drugs.

Guaifenesin. rINN for GUAIPHENESIN.

Guaiphenesin. Used to reduce sputum viscosity.

Guanethidine. Adrenergic neurone blocking drug. Used in hypertension. Eye drops used in glaucoma and hyperthyroid eye signs. Adverse effects include postural hypotension, nasal stuffiness, diarrhoea, fluid retention, and impotence. Action antagonized by tricyclic antidepressants and sympathomimetics (e.g., when used as nasal decongestants in 'cold cures').

Guanochlor. Antihypertensive adrenergic neurone blocking drug with actions similar to GUANETHIDINE.

Guanoxan. Antihypertensive adrenergic neurone blocking drug with actions similar to GUANETHIDINE.

Guar flour. *See* GUAR GUM.

Guar gum. Binding agent in tablets, thickening agent in foods. Takes in moisture from the gut and produces feeling of satiety by the bulk thus formed. Used in treatment of obesity and in diabetes mellitus where it may help to stabilize blood glucose levels. Unwanted effects include abdominal bloating, indigestion, diarrhoea, and flatus.

H

Haemophilus influenza type b vaccine. Vaccine prepared from the purified polysaccharide of the capsule of the Haemophilus influenza type b virus, conjugated with the tetanus protein (Act-HIB) or diphtheria protein (Hib-TITER) to increase its effectiveness and duration of protection. Recommended for general vaccination programmes in infants over 2 months of age to reduce incidence of childhood meningitis due to this organism. Local skin redness may occur at the injection site.

Halcinonide. Topical CORTICOSTEROID used in psoriasis and eczema.

Halofantrine. Antimalarial effective in acute treatment of infections resistant to CHLOROQUINE, and other antimalarials. May cause gastro-intestinal disturbances and potentially fatal cardiac arrhythmias. Also a risk of fatal arrhythmias if given together with mefloquine or other drugs which may induce arrhythmias or electrolyte imbalance. Fatty foods may increase absorption and should therefore be avoided.

Haloperidol. Butyrophenone tranquillizer. Used in treatment of psychosis where it has similar effects to CHLORPROMAZINE but more potent. Has antiemetic action but lacks anticholinergic and alpha-adrenolytic effects. May cause involuntary movements, drowsiness, depression, hypotension, sweating, skin reactions, and jaundice. In overdosage effects and treatment similar to CHLORPROMAZINE.

Halopyramine. Antihistamine similar to PROMETHAZINE.

Halothane. Potent inhalational anaesthetic used for major surgery. Adverse effects include slowing of the heart and fall in blood pressure. May cause liver damage with jaundice in susceptible patients on repeated exposure.

Heparin, low molecular weight. Prepared by fractionating naturally occuring HEPARIN. Shares some of the properties and actions of standard HEPARIN but has a longer duration of action and is less likely to cause bleeding and other side effects.

Heparin. Anticoagulant produced in mast cells and obtained from bovine lung. Acts by preventing several reactions in the blood-clotting mechanism. Given by injection only. Used to prevent formation or spread of blood clots as in deep vein thrombosis of the legs or heart valve prostheses. May produce allergic reactions and, on prolonged use, osteoporosis. Heparin-induced haemorrhage may be controlled by PROTAMINE SULPHATE. Low molecular weight heparins are prepared by fractionating naturally occurring HEPARIN. They share some of the properties and actions of standard HEPARIN but have a longer duration of action and are less likely to cause bleeding and other side effects.

Heparinoid. Heparin derivative or similar substance with uses and effects similar to HEPARIN.

Hepatitis A vaccine. Vaccine prepared from purified inactivated viral antigens for protection against transmissible viral hepatitis. Used in high risk groups (e.g.

health care personnel). Adverse effects include fever, malaise, nausea, loss of appetite, soreness at injection site.

Hepatitis B vaccine. Vaccine prepared from purified inactivated viral antigens for protection against transmissible viral hepatitis. Used in 'at risk' populations (e.g., health-care personnel and drug abusers). Adverse effects include fever, joint pains, nausea, tiredness, and rashes.

Heroin (c). *See* DIAMORPHINE.

Hetastarch. Polysaccharide used intravenously instead of blood or plasma to maintain blood volume.

Hexachlorophane. Topical antiseptic used in soaps, creams, lotions, and dusting powders. Adverse effects include allergy, light sensitivity, and CNS effects if absorbed or ingested.

Hexamethonium. Ganglion-blocking drug used parenterally in hypertension. Adverse effects include postural hypotension, dry mouth, paralysis of accommodation, retention of urine, constipation, and impotence.

Hexamine. Antiseptic used topically and for urinary infections. For the latter use, the urine must be rendered acid by also giving AMMONIUM CHLORIDE which liberates formaldehyde from the hexamine. May cause painful micturition, frequency, and haematuria.

Hexamine mandelate. Compound of HEXAMINE and MANDELIC ACID, used as urinary antiseptic. Requires acid urine. Adverse effects include nausea and vomiting.

Hexetidine. Topical antibacterial/antifungal/antitrichomonas.

Hexobarbitone (c). Barbiturate hypnotic essentially like AMYLOBARBITONE.

Hexylresorcinol. Antiworm. Also used as antiseptic agent for throat infections.

Histamine. Mediator of many body functions including gastric secretion, inflammatory and allergic responses. Produces skin vasodilation. Was used in test of gastric acid production. Adverse effects include headache, hypotension, bronchospasm, and diarrhoea.

Homatropine. Parasympatholytic with actions, toxic effects, etc. similar to ATROPINE. Used as a mydriatic because when compared with ATROPINE its action is more rapid, less prolonged, and more easily reversed by PHYSOSTIGMINE.

Human menopausal gonadotrophins. Preparation containing human follicle stimulating hormone and luteinizing hormone used to treat infertility due to failure of gonadotrophin stimulation, by stimulating ovulation in women and sperm production in men. Should not be used in other causes of infertility. May cause allergic reactions including skin rashes.

Hyaluronidase. Enzyme that assists dispersal and absorption of subcutaneous and intramuscular injections. Hastens resorption of blood and fluid in body cavities. Adverse effects include allergic reactions.

Hydralazine. Vasodilator antihypertensive drug. Adverse effects include tachycardia, headache, marrow depression, acute rheumatoid syndrome, and systemic lupus erythematosus syndrome.

Hydrochlorothiazide. Thiazide diuretic similar to BENDROFLUAZIDE.

Hydrocortisone. Naturally occurring adrenocorticosteroid hormone with similar actions, etc. to CORTISONE.

Hydroflumethiazide. Thiazide diuretic similar to BENDROFLUAZIDE.

Hydrogen peroxide. Disinfectant/deodorant. Acts by rapid but short-lived release of oxygen. Used for cleaning wounds. Also helps to detach dead tissue. Other uses include mouth wash, treatment of acne and minor skin infections, and bleaching hair.

Hydromorphone. Opioid analgesic with greater potency than MORPHINE but with similar adverse effects. Used by injection in the management of moderate to severe pain.

Hydrotalcite. Antacid used in peptic ulcer and gastric hyperacidity.

Hydrous wool fat. Purified waxy substance obtained from the wool of sheep plus water. Used as a base for ointments. May produce skin sensitization.

Hydroxocobalamin (Vitamin B_{12}). Used for the treatment of pernicious anaemia or specific deficiency states. Parenteral.

Hydroxyapatite. Calcium salt used as a source of calcium and phosphorus in osteoporosis, rickets, and osteomalacia.

Hydroxycarbamide. rINN for HYDROXYUREA.

Hydroxychloroquine. Antimalarial agent: *see* CHLOROQUINE.

Hydroxyprogesterone. Actions and uses similar to PROGESTERONE.

Hydroxyquinoline. Topical antibacterial/antifungal deodorant.

5-Hydroxytryptamine. Neurotransmitter with central and peripheral actions. Thought to be involved in the vascular headache of migraine and to be deficient in some types of depression.

Hydroxyurea. Cytotoxic agent for oral administration.

Hydroxyzine. CNS depressant. Used to relieve tension and anxiety in emotional disturbances but less effective than CHLORPROMAZINE and similar tranquillizers in the psychoses. May cause excessive drowsiness, headache, dry mouth, itching, and convulsions. Coma in overdosage. No antidote; supportive treatment only.

Hyoscine butylbromide. Parasympatholytic, with peripheral actions similar to ATROPINE SULPHATE but of shorter duration. Used as an antispasmodic similar to PROPANTHELINE but effective only by injection.

Hyoscine hydrobromide. Parasympatholytic, with central and peripheral actions similar to ATROPINE SULPHATE except that it produces central depression and hypnosis rather than stimulation and that it tends to slow the heart. Used for pre-operative medication where the hypnotic effect makes it preferable to atropine and as an antiemetic for travel sickness. Adverse effects, etc. otherwise as for ATROPINE SULPHATE.

Hyoscine methobromide. Similar to HYOSCINE HYDROBROMIDE.

Hypromellose. Indigestible plant residue similar to METHYLCELLULOSE but used mainly in eye drops as lubricant (e.g., in so-called artificial tears for dry eyes).

I

Ibuprofen. Non-steroid anti-inflammatory/analgesic/antipyretic. Reduces inflammation by inhibition of prostaglandin synthesis, which is part of the inflammatory process. Used in rheumatoid arthritis and other arthritic conditions. Used also as a general purpose mild analgesic and as an antipyretic in febrile conditions of childhood. Also inhibits prostaglandin synthesis in gastric mucosa, thus reducing their protective effect and causing gastric intolerance. Gastro-intestinal symptoms, including blood loss, are less common than with ASPIRIN. Other adverse effects include headache, other CNS symptoms and hypersensitivity reactions.

Ichthammol. Dermatological preparation, with slight antibacterial effects. Used in creams and ointments for chronic skin conditions.

Icodextrin. Non-absorbable glucose polymer used in ambulatory peritoneal dialysis as treatment of end-stage chronic renal failure. Avoids the weight gain and high glucose/insulin levels associated with dialysis solution based on glucose. May cause abdominal pain, muscle cramps, fluid and electrolyte imbalance.

Idarubicin. Cytotoxic antibiotic with actions, uses and adverse effects similar to DAUNORUBICIN.

Idoxuridine. Antiviral agent used in local treatment of herpes infections.

Ifosfamide. Cytotoxic drug, with uses and adverse effects similar to CYCLOPHOSPHAMIDE.

Imipenem. Intravenous broad-spectrum antibiotic which acts by inhibiting bacterial cell wall synthesis, similar to PENICILLINS and CEPHALOSPORINS. Active against many penicillin-resistant strains. Given in combination with CILASTATIN, a structurally similar compound with no antibacterial activity which helps to reduce the metabolism of imipenem and thus to prolong its effectiveness. Adverse effects include nausea, vomiting, diarrhoea, blood dyscrasias and disturbance of renal, hepatic and CNS functions. May cross-react in patients with PENICILLIN hypersensitivity.

Imipramine. Antidepressant, blocks neuronal re-uptake of NORADRENALINE, DOPAMINE, and 5-HYDROXYTRYPTAMINE. Adverse effects include anticholinergic actions of dry mouth, blurred vision, precipitation of glaucoma, retention of urine, and constipation; also produces cardiac arrhythmias, potentiates direct sympathomimetic pressor amines and antagonizes action of GUANETHIDINE, BETHANIDINE, DEBRISOQUINE and CLONIDINE. Coma, convulsions and cardiac arrhythmias in overdosage. Treatment supportive.

Immunoglobulin G. Concentrate of antibodies derived from human plasma. Used to convey short-term immunity to some virus infections including hepatitis A, measles and rubella. Used in cases of congenital and acquired immunoglobulin deficiency and after bone marrow transplantation.

Inactivated lactobacilli. Vaccine from bacteria found in the vagina of women suffering from trichomonal infection. The vaccine provokes the immune response to infections including trichomoniasis and thus helps to prevent recurrent infections.

Indapamide. Derivative of FRUSEMIDE, used as antihypertensive in subdiuretic doses. Larger doses have diuretic action and adverse effects similar to BENDROFLUAZIDE.

Indinavir. Antiviral with activity against HIV. Used in combination with other antiviral agents as prophylaxis in immunodeficient patients with AIDS. May cause gastro-intestinal disturbance, skin reactions, muscle pains and numbness.

Indometacin. rINN for INDOMETHACIN.

Indomethacin. Non-steroid anti-inflammatory/analgesic, used in treatment of inflammatory joint disease. Adverse effects include headache, vertigo, depression, confusion, and gastro-intestinal symptoms including perforation and haemorrhage.

Indoprofen. Non-steroid anti-inflammatory/analgesic, with actions, uses, and adverse effects similar to IBUPROFEN. Recently withdrawn.

Indoramin. Alpha-adrenoceptor blocking drug, used in hypertension, peripheral vascular disease, prophylaxis of migraine and symptomatic relief of urinary symptoms due to prostatic hypertrophy. Acts by relaxation of muscles in blood vessels and in prostate gland. Produces sedation and nasal stuffiness.

Inosine pranobex. Antiviral active against herpes simplex in skin and mucous membranes. Used for genital warts. Does not act directly against the virus, but increases the body's cellular immune response. Metabolized to uric acid and thus may cause elevated uric acid levels. Caution if used in gout or renal failure.

Inositol. Ingredient of nutritional preparations. It has been considered a vitamin but no nutritional deficiency has been demonstrated.

Inositol nicotinate. Metabolized to nicotinic acid which dilates peripheral blood vessels. Used for chilblains and other conditions where peripheral blood circulation is thought to be poor. Large doses may cause fall in blood pressure and slowing of heart.

Insulin. Hormone. Available as pig or beef insulin derived from animal pancreas and as human insulin now available by synthesis from animal insulin or by genetic engineering from bacterial sources. Causes a fall in blood sugar levels and increased storage of glycogen in the liver. Used parenterally to treat diabetes. Different formulations are produced to provide varied duration of action. Adverse effects include hypoglycaemia and subcutaneous fat atrophy.

Interferon alpha-2a. Antiviral agent produced from bacteria by recombinant techniques (genetic engineering). Used to suppress growth of the AIDS-related Kaposi's sarcoma, chronic myelogenous leukaemia, 'hairy cell' leukaemia, and chronic active hepatitis. May cause 'flu-like syndrome, anorexia, weight loss and effects on the CNS and cardiovascular system. Less likely to cause further suppression of immune system than conventional cytotoxics, but full monitoring is needed.

Interferon alpha-2b. Antiviral agent similar to INTERFERON ALPHA-2A but, at present, used for treatment of 'hairy cell' leukaemia and non-Hodgkin's lymphoma, chronic myelogenous leukaemia, malignant melanoma, and chronic active hepatitis. Further trials may extend its use to other cancers. Adverse effects similar to those from Interferon alpha-2a, but may include bleeding.

Interferon alpha-NI. Antiviral agent with actions and adverse effects similar to INTERFERON ALPHA–2B at present used only for treatment of 'hairy cell' leukaemia, but under investigation for use in other cancers. May also cause liver and kidney damage.

Interferon beta-1a and Interferon beta-1b. Genetically engineered proteins with actions which reduce immune mechanisms. Used to reduce or prevent relapses in multiple sclerosis although the exact mechanism of action is not known. May cause influenza-like symptoms, pain at the injection site and CNS effects including convulsions.

Interferon gamma. Used as adjunctive therapy to antibiotics in patients with the rare condition chronic granulomatous disease, in which there is reduced resistance to infection. Produced by biotechnology, it is identical to a human substance involved in resisting infection. Unwanted effects include fever, muscle and joint pains.

Iodine. Halogen, converted to iodide in the body and used in production of thyroid hormone. Low dietary intake leads to reduced thyroid function (myxoedema). Large doses may be given by mouth to suppress thyroid function prior to surgical removal of thyroid tissue when the gland is overactive. May cause hypersensitivity with headache, laryngitis, bronchitis, and rashes. May also be used on the skin as a disinfectant.

Ipecacuanha. Plant extract used in small doses as an expectorant in cough mixtures. Emetic effect if larger doses (syrup of ipecacuanha) are used in children as emergency treatment of ingested poisons.

Ipratropium. Anticholinergic used by inhalation for its bronchodilator action in chronic bronchitis and asthma. Used also as intranasal spray for relief of chronic watery nasal discharge. Adverse effects similar to ATROPINE, but much reduced when given by inhalation and are seen only at high doses.

Iprindol. Antidepressant, with actions, uses, and adverse effects similar to IMIPRAMINE.

Irbesartan. Antihypertensive. ANGIOTENSIN II receptor antagonist with actions, uses and adverse effects similar to LOSARTAN.

Irinotecan. Cytotoxic used in treatment of metastatic colorectal cancer in patients resistant to 5-FLUOROURACIL. It is a prodrug that is converted to two active metabolites which inhibit DNA replication. May cause nausea, vomiting, bone marrow suppression and "delayed diarrhoea" 24 hours or more after treatment. This condition could be life threatening and requires hospital treatment.

Iron dextran injection. Parenteral formulation for iron-deficiency anaemia. Adverse effects include pain on injection, skin staining, vomiting, headache, and dizziness. Anaphylactic reactions may accompany intravenous infusion particularly.

Iron sorbitol injection. Intramuscular formulation for iron deficiency anaemia. Adverse effects as for IRON DEXTRAN INJECTION.

Isoaminile citrate. Cough suppressant used on its own or in cough linctus. No analgesic or sedative effects. Does not depress respiration. May cause dizziness, nausea, and constipation or diarrhoea.

Isocarboxazid. Monoamine oxidase inhibitor/antidepressant. Actions, uses, and adverse effects as for PHENELZINE.

Isoconazole. Used to treat fungal and protozoal vaginal infections. Actions and adverse effects similar to METRONIDAZOLE.

Isoflurane. Potent inhalational anaesthetic used for major surgery. Has also analgesic properties. More potent than HALOTHANE in depressing respiration and enhancing effects of muscle relaxants (e.g., TUBOCURARINE) but less likely to sensitize the heart to catecholamines.

Isometheptene. Sympathomimetic agent, with actions and adverse effects similar to ADRENALINE. Used in symptomatic treatment of migraine where it is said to constrict the dilated blood vessels that cause the throbbing headache.

Isoniazid. Synthetic anti-tuberculous agent. About 60 percent of Caucasians are slow inactivators by acetylation, genetically determined. Adverse effects include peripheral neuropathy, pellagra, mental disturbances, and convulsions, which may be reduced by administration of PYRIDOXINE.

Isoprenaline. Beta-adrenoceptor agonist used in bronchial asthma by inhalation or orally. Adverse effects include tachycardia, arrhythmias, and tremor. May also be used as intravenous infusion in treatment of shock. More likely to cause cardiac arrhythmias than DOPAMINE or DOBUTAMINE.

Isosorbide dinitrate (Sorbide nitrate). Dilates blood vessels. Similar actions and adverse effects to GLYCERYL TRINITRATE but longer action. Used for symptomatic and prophylactic treatment of angina and in resistant heart failure.

Isosorbide mononitrate. Vasodilator used for prophylaxis of angina. An active metabolite of ISOSORBIDE DINITRATE, it is not metabolized further and may thus have a more predictable effect. Adverse effects are similar to GLYCERYL TRINITRATE.

Isotretinoin. Vitamin A derivative, used to treat severe acne not responsive to antibiotic therapy. Thought to act directly on sebaceous glands in the skin to reduce sebum production. Adverse effects include dryness of skin, mucous membranes and conjunctivae. Teratogenesis, nausea, headache, malaise, joint pains, hair loss, and biochemical evidence of liver damage may also occur. Contraindicated in the presence of liver or kidney disease, in pregnancy or in patients with a history or family history of cutaneous epithelioma. Local irritation may occur after topical application. Has been associated with depression.

Ispaghula. Purgative. Dried, ripe seeds of *Plantago ovata.* Increases faecal bulk. Mechanism of action similar to that of METHYLCELLULOSE.

Ispaghula husk. As for ISPAGHULA, but contains only outer layers of dried seeds and is more potent than whole seeds. Also used as an adjunct to diet, for its ability to lower blood cholesterol concentrations by removing cholesterol and fatty acids from the gut. May cause flatulence and bloating.

Isradipine. Antihypertensive which lowers blood pressure by dilating blood vessels. Adverse reactions include headache, flushing, dizziness, tachycardia, palpitations, localized peripheral oedema, weight gain, fatigue and abdominal discomfort. Similar in action to NIFEDIPINE.

Itraconazole. Antifungal agent for oral treatment of vulvovaginal candidiasis, pityriasis versicolor and dermatophytoses. May cause nausea, dyspepsia, abdominal pain and headache.

K

Kanamycin. Bactericidal aminoglycoside antibiotic with actions and spectrum similar to NEOMYCIN, but less ototoxic. Used in gram-negative septicaemia, with monitoring of blood levels, particularly in renal failure. Potentiates neuromuscular blockade.

Kaolin. Adsorbent. Used externally as a dusting powder and by mouth as treatment for diarrhoea where it increases faecal bulk and slows passage through the gut. Once thought to have specific adsorbent effect for poisonous substances but it is now known that the adsorbent effect is a general one.

Ketamine (m). Parenteral anaesthetic with analgesic properties in subanaesthetic doses. Rapid onset of action, but may cause psychotic symptoms, including hallucinations, the frequency of which can be reduced by giving DIAZEPAM or DROPERIDOL. Contraindicated in patients with high blood pressure or known psychosis.

Ketoconazole. Used to treat internal and external fungal infections. Adverse effects include nausea, rashes, and jaundice.

Ketoprofen. Anti-inflammatory/analgesic, with actions, uses and adverse effects similar to IBUPROFEN.

Ketorolac. Non-steroidal anti-inflammatory analgesic with actions similar to IBUPROFEN. Used intramuscularly or orally to relieve post-operative pain. May cause pain at injection site, drowsiness, sweating and gastro-intestinal symptoms. Dose and duration of use restricted because of severity of gastro-intestinal effects, asthma and anaphylaxis. May also be used topically as eye drops following eye surgery.

Ketotifen. Preventative treatment for asthma. Has the actions of an antihistamine, similar to PROMETHAZINE and also blocks allergic mechanisms by a mechanism similar to SODIUM CROMOGLYCATE. Adverse effects include dry mouth, dizziness, and sedation.

L

Labetalol. Antihypertensive. Has both alpha- and beta-adrenoceptor blocking actions. Uses and adverse effects similar to PROPRANOLOL. Postural hypotension may occur.

Lachesine. Parasympatholytic, similar to TROPICAMIDE. Used in the eye as a mydriatic and cycloplegic.

Lacidipine. Calcium channel antagonist used to treat hypertension. Mode of action and adverse reactions similar to NIFEDIPINE but used only once daily.

Lactic acid. Used intravenously as dilute solution in treatment of acidosis. Acts less rapidly than SODIUM BICARBONATE. Also used topically as strong solutions in treatment of warts.

Lactitol. A semi-synthetic disaccharide consisting of galatose and sorbitol, with actions and uses similar to LACTULOSE.

Lactulose. Laxative. A synthetic disaccharide (galactose plus fructose) that is not absorbed but broken down by gut bacteria to nonabsorbable products that increase the faecal mass by osmotic effects. Effective but expensive. Has been recommended for use in liver failure to reduce absorption of ammonia from the gut.

Laevodopa. *See* LEVODOPA.

Laevulose. Carbohydrate. Used intravenously as a source of calories when oral feeding is not possible. In renal failure it is better tolerated than dextrose. Accelerates metabolism of ethyl alcohol and may be used to treat alcohol poisoning. May cause facial flushing, abdominal pain, and localized thrombophlebitis.

Lamivudine. Antiviral agent active against HIV. Used in combination with other antivirals in progressive disease (AIDS). May cause gastro-intestinal disturbance, muscle and joint pains and bone marrow suppression. Acts synergistically with ZIDOVUDINE and these drugs may be used in combination.

Lamotrigine. Anticonvulsant. Acts by inhibiting excitatory neurotransmitter release and by stabilizing neuronal membranes. Can be used alone or as a second-line, additional treatment in patients not satisfactorily controlled on other anticonvulsants. May cause drowsiness, headache, blurred vision, gastrointestinal disturbances and skin rashes.

Lanolin. Purified, fat-like substance from the wool of sheep. Used in creams for topical use, it is not absorbed but aids the absorption of drugs carried in the cream. Otherwise used for its emulsifying effect in bland creams and cosmetics. May cause skin sensitization.

Lanreotide. Long-acting analogue of the growth hormone releasing hormone (somatostatin). Used by fortnightly injections to treat acromegaly. May cause pain at injection site, gastro-intestinal upset and gallstones.

Lansoprazole. Suppresses production of gastric acid. Actions, uses and adverse effects similar to OMEPRAZOLE.

L-Asparaginase (Colaspase). Cytotoxic enzyme derived from bacterial culture; used in neoplastic disease. Adverse effects include nausea, vomiting, pyrexia, neurotoxicity, hypersensitivity reactions, and bone marrow depression.

Latanoprost. Prostaglandin analogue which increases fluid outflow from the anterior chamber of the eye, thus reducing intra-occular pressure. Used as eye drops in the treatment of glaucoma. May cause eye discomfort, reddening and blurred vision.

LAX (levo-acetyl-3,4 methylenedioxyphenyliosprenaline hydrochloride) (m). An illicit drug derivative abused for its euphoriant and hallucinogenic effects. Said to be derived from MDMA.

L-**Dopa.** *See* LEVODOPA.

Lecithins. Phospholipids found in both animal and vegetable foods. Used as emulsifying and stabilizing agents in skin preparations.

Lenograstim. Closely related to FILGRASTIM, and sharing the same indications. Adverse effects include bone pain and local reactions at the injection site.

Lepirudin. Genetically engineered anticoagulant with actions similar to hirudin, the anticoagulant found in leeches. Acts to prevent clot formation at several stages without the need for co-factors. Used to treat HEPARIN-associated thrombocytopaenia which is characterised by formation of life-threatening blood clots. May cause bleeding, fever and renal failure.

Lercanidipine. Long-acting calcium antagonist with actions similar to NIFEDEPINE. Used as a once-daily treatment for hypertension. May cause flushing, peripheral oedema and headache.

Letrozole. Antioestrogen. Acts by inhibiting enzymes controlling oestrogen production. Used in treatment of advanced breast cancer in patients in whom TAMOXIFEN has failed. Adverse effects include headache, nausea, tiredness, cough and hot flushes.

Leuprorelin. An analogue of gonadotrophin releasing hormone which initially increases but then suppresses sex hormone production. Used to reduce growth of cancer of the prostate and before surgery of the uterus. May cause initial transient increase in bone pain and urinary obstruction and later, loss of libido, hot flushes and sweating.

Levallorphan. Narcotic antagonist similar to NALORPHINE. Less likely to cause severe withdrawal symptoms in 'addicts'.

Levamisole. Antiworm treatment. Used mainly in veterinary practice but also in man against *Ascaris* sp. (roundworm). Adverse effects include nausea, vomiting, abdominal pain, and fall in blood pressure.

Levobunolol. A non-selective beta-adrenoceptor blocker formulated as eyedrops to treat glaucoma by lowering intraocular pressure. Actions and adverse effects similar to TIMOLOL and PROPRANOLOL.

Levocabastine. Antihistamine, potent blocker of H_1. Used topically as nasal spray and eye drops to reduce the symptoms of hay fever (allergic rhinitis/conjunctivitis). May cause local irritation, blurred vision, headache and tiredness.

Levodopa. Amino acid. Converted in body to DOPAMINE, a neurotransmitter substance that is deficient in Parkinson's disease. Controls rigidity and improves movements but less effect on tremor than anticholinergic drugs (e.g., BENZHEXOL). May cause gastro-intestinal symptoms, hypotension, involuntary movements, and psychiatric disturbances. Side effects may be reduced by combination with peripheral inhibitors of dopamine synthesis (e.g., CARBIDOPA). Contraindicated/caution in cardiovascular disease and psychiatric disturbance. Effects diminished by phenothiazines (e.g., CHLORPROMAZINE), METHYLDOPA, RESERPINE, PYRIDOXINE.

Levofloxacin. Antibiotic with actions, uses and adverse effects similar to CIPROFLOXACIN.

Levomepromazine. rINN for METHOTRIMEPRAZINE.

Levonorgestrel. *See* NORGESTREL.

Levonorgestrel. Sex hormone with actions, uses and adverse effects similar to PROGESTERONE. Also used topically through an intrauterine contraceptive device, when adverse reactions include altered menstrual patterns, lower abdominal pain and back pain.

Levorphanol (c). Narcotic analgesic similar to MORPHINE, but more reliable when given by mouth. Useful in the management of severe chronic pain in terminal disease.

Levothyroxine. rINN for THYROXINE.

Lidocaine. rINN for LIGNOCAINE.

Lignocaine. Local anaesthetic/antiarrhythmic. Stabilizes nerve cell membranes to prevent impulse conduction. Used topically or by injection for local anaesthesia in minor operations. Intravenous injection or infusion used to treat abnormal heart rhythms. Excessive doses also block motor impulses and normal cardiac conduction. May cause hypotension, CNS depression and convulsions. Metabolized by liver and therefore used with caution in liver disease. Short action prevents use as oral antiarrhythmic.

Lindane. Organochlorine insecticide. Used topically on skin/hair for lice and scabies. Safe, providing not ingested, but emergence of resistant strains of the parasites limits its effectiveness.

Liothyronine. Thyroid hormone, probably the active hormone to which THYROXINE is converted. Given by mouth or injection it has effects similar to THYROXINE but more rapid and short-lived. Used when rapid effect is needed (e.g., in myxoedema coma). Used with care if there is evidence of cardiovascular disease as it may precipitate cardiac failure.

Liquid paraffin. Laxative. Lubricates faecal material in colon and rectum. Used when straining is undesirable or defaecation painful (e.g., after operations for haemorrhoids). Reduces absorption of fat-soluble VITAMIN A and VITAMIN D, and in chronic use can cause paraffinomas in mesenteric lymph glands. May leak from anal sphincter. Also used in some topical skin and eye preparations as a lubricant and an aid to removal of crusts.

Liquorice. Dried plant root with expectorant and mild anti-inflammatory properties. Used as a flavouring/expectorant in cough mixtures. DEGLYCYRRHIZINISED LIQUORICE is used in treatment of peptic ulceration. Large doses may cause salt and water retention leading to hypertension and/or cardiac failure.

Lisinopril. Antihypertensive, with actions, uses and adverse effects similar to CAPTOPRIL.

Lisuride. rINN for LYSURIDE.

Lithium salts. Usually given as carbonate or citrate, provides lithium ions which substitute for sodium in excitable tissues and reduce brain catecholamine levels. Used in prophylactic treatment of mania and depression. Caution in cardiac or renal disease. Needs careful control of plasma levels. Adverse effects include tremor, vomiting, diarrhoea, ataxia, blurred vision, thirst, polyuria leading to confusion and fits, and coma in gross overdosage. Lithium excretion may be enhanced by forced alkaline diuresis, peritoneal dialysis, or haemodialysis. Intoxication may be precipitated by diuretic therapy or salt restriction. Lithium succinate has anti-inflammatory and antifungal activity and is used as topical treatment for seborrhoeic dermatitis. It may cause skin irritation but does not have systemic effects.

Liver extracts. Extracts of liver prepared for oral use were used for treatment of pernicious anaemia. Unpalatable and irregularly absorbed. Now replaced by the pure vitamin B_{12} (HYDROXOCOBALAMIN).

Lodoxamide. Anti-allergic, used in treatment of allergic conjunctivitis by topical ocular application. It has actions similar to SODIUM CROMOGLYCATE.

Lofepramine. Antidepressant, metabolized to DESIPRAMINE, after absorption. Actions, uses, and adverse effects similar to AMITRIPTYLINE.

Lofexidine. Central-acting alpha receptor agonist with actions similar to CLONIDINE. Used in the supportive treatment of withdrawal from opiate addiction where it suppresses the noradrenergic symptoms of withdrawal (e.g., sweating, diarrhoea, muscle cramps). Unlike CLONIDINE is less likely to cause sedation at the doses needed. May cause dry mouth and drowsiness, and could exacerbate existing cardiovascular disease.

Lomustine (CCNU). Cytotoxic drug used in neoplastic disease. Adverse effects include loss of appetite, nausea, vomiting, liver toxicity, and bone marrow depression.

Loperamide. Antidiarrhoeal, with actions, uses, and adverse effects similar to DIPHENOXYLATE.

Loprazolam. Benzodiazepine, used for short-term treatment of insomnia. Actions and adverse effects similar to DIAZEPAM.

Loratadine. Antihistamine with long duration of action, suitable for once-daily dosing. Similar to AZATADINE, but claimed to produce less sedation.

Lorazepam. Benzodiazepine anxiolytic similar to DIAZEPAM.

Losartan. Selective angiotensin II antagonist with effects similar to angiotensin-converting enzyme (ACE) inhibitors e.g. CAPTOPRIL, but more selective. Used as an antihypertensive where it does not cause dry cough or the allergic reactions associated with ACE inhibitors. May cause dizziness and rashes. Compared to ACE inhibitors this class of drugs appear safer to use in patients with impaired renal function.

Loxapine. Antipsychotic with similar effects to phenothiazines such as CHLORPROMAZINE but chemically different, and less likely to produce extrapyramidal side effects. Adverse effects include dizziness, faintness, muscle twitching, weakness and confusion, peristent tardive dyskinesia, tachycardia, hypo- or hypertension, ECG changes, skin reactions, anticholinergic effects, nausea, vomiting, dyspnoea, and headache.

LSD (Lysergic acid diethylamide) (m). Hallucinogen. Not used therapeutically but abused for its psychedelic effects – notably altered visual perception. Consciousness and awareness not altered, but may cause thought disorders, personality changes and apparent psychotic disease. Other 'unwanted' effects include gastro-intestinal disturbance, sweating, and incoordination. Delayed 'flashback' adverse effects may occur even months after use and especially in the presence of stress or other CNS active drugs. Causes tolerance but not physical dependence.

Lymecycline. Bacteriostatic antibiotic, with actions, adverse effects, and interactions similar to TETRACYCLINE.

Lynoestrenol. Sex hormone (progestogen) with actions, uses, and adverse effects similar to NORETHISTERONE.

Lypressin. Hormone extract from posterior pituitary gland of pigs. Actions, uses, and adverse effects similar to VASOPRESSIN.

Lysergic acid diethylamide. *See* LSD.

Lysergide. *See* LSD.

Lysine. Essential AMINO ACID also used as a buffer to reduce acidity/gastric irritation from ACETYL SALICYLIC ACID.

Lysuride. Dopamine agonist with actions and adverse effects similar to BROMOCRIPTINE. Used in Parkinson's disease where it may add to the effects of LEVODOPA, especially in later stages of the disease when treatment is failing.

M

Magaldrate. Antacid. Complex hydrated form of MAGNESIUM SULPHATE and aluminium sulphate.

Magnesium alginate. Magnesium salt of ALGINIC ACID, used as emulsifying/thickening agent in antacid preparations for treatment of acid reflux.

Magnesium antacids. Range of magnesium salts used alone or complexed with other compounds. Neutralize gastric acid in treatment of peptic ulceration. Large doses have laxative effect which may be reduced by combination with ALUMINIUM ANTACIDS. Very little absorbed but danger of toxic magnesium blood levels in renal failure. May reduce absorption of other drugs (e.g., TETRACYCLINES).

Magnesium carbonate. Nonsystemic antacid with similar actions, uses, and adverse effects to MAGNESIUM HYDROXIDE. Releases carbon dioxide in stomach and may cause belching.

Magnesium citrate. Osmotic purgative. Solution used to aid removal or prevent formation of crystals in long-term urinary catheterization.

Magnesium hydroxide. Nonsystemic antacid (only 10 percent absorbed). Used in treatment of peptic ulceration. Neutralizes gastric acid and acts longer than SODIUM BICARBONATE. May have laxative effect, which can be prevented by simultaneous use of ALUMINIUM ANTACIDS.

Magnesium oxide. Nonsystemic antacid. Converted to MAGNESIUM HYDROXIDE in the stomach and has similar actions and adverse effects.

Magnesium sulphate (Epsom salts). Osmotic purgative. Absorbed only slowly from gut. Magnesium and sulphate ions attract or retain water by osmosis and thus increase bulk of intestinal contents. Effective in three to six hours. Produces semi-fluid or watery stools, therefore useful as single treatment but not for repeated dosage. Danger of systemic toxicity from magnesium in patients with reduced renal function.

Magnesium trisilicate. Nonsystemic antacid used in treatment of peptic ulceration. Neutralization of acid is slow in onset but relatively prolonged due to adsorbent properties of silicic acid formed in the stomach. Has a laxative effect in larger doses. Danger of magnesium toxicity in patients with renal failure.

Malathion. Organophosphorus insecticide. Acts by inhibition of cholinesterase and may therefore produce toxic effects due to accumulation of excess ACETYLCHOLINE. One of the least toxic of this group of insecticides, low concentrations of malathion may be used on human skin for infestation (e.g., lice) without systemic effects. Toxic effects may be treated by antidotes ATROPINE SULPHATE and PRALIDOXIME.

Malic acid. Found in apples and pears. Formerly used in tooth-cleaning tablets. Used as part of an astringent skin treatment.

Mandelic acid. Excreted unchanged in the urine where it has antibacterial (bacteriostatic) actions. Used orally in combination with HEXAMINE as HEXAMINE MANDELATE. May also be instilled directly into the bladder during prolonged use of urinary catheters.

Manganese. Trace element sometimes added to nutritional preparations for supposed increase in the haematinic effects of iron.

Manganese sulphate. Occasionally used as a haematinic. Said to increase the effect of FERROUS SULPHATE in treatment of iron-deficiency anaemia.

Mannitol. Osmotic diuretic. Opposes reabsorption of water which normally accompanies sodium reabsorption from kidney tubule. Used when there is danger of renal failure (e.g., shock, cardiovascular surgery) and in fluid overload refractory to other diuretics. May cause cardiac failure owing to increased circulating blood volume.

Maprotiline. Antidepressant, with actions, uses, and adverse effects similar to IMIPRAMINE.

Mazindol (c). Anorectic indole derivative with central stimulant properties. Produces tachycardia and rise in blood pressure.

MDA (Methoxydesmethylamphetamine) (m). Amphetamine derivative similar to MDMA.

MDEA (Methoxydesethylamphetamine) (m). Amphetamine derivative similar to MDMA.

MDMA (Methylenedioxymethamphetamine) (m). Amphetamine derivative abused for its euphoriant and hallucinogenic effects. Although thought by users to be safe, when used at dance parties (raves), the combination of excessive exercise and dehydration has been associated with hyperpyrexia, heat stroke and death.

Measles vaccine. Live attenuated measles virus for measles immunization. Adverse effects include mild fever, rash, and rare neurological disorders. Use with care if there is a history of convulsions or epilepsy.

Mebendazole. Used in treatment of roundworm. Actions and adverse effects as for THIABENDAZOLE.

Mebeverine. Antispasmodic, with direct action on colonic smooth muscle but no systemic anticholinergic effects. Used for relief of abdominal pain and cramps (e.g., due to irritable colon or non-specific diarrhoea).

Mecysteine. rINN for METHYLCYSTEINE.

Medazepam. Benzodiazepine anxiolytic similar to DIAZEPAM but with less anticonvulsant activity. Used in the treatment of anxiety.

Medigoxin. Actions, uses, and adverse effects similar to DIGOXIN.

Medium-chain triglycerides. A mixture of triglycerides from straight-chain fatty acids for use in fat malabsorption syndromes.

Medroxyprogesterone. Sex hormone, with actions and adverse effects similar to PROGESTERONE. Used to treat hormone-dependent malignancies (e.g., of breast, endometrium and prostate).

Mefenamic acid. Anti-inflammatory/analgesic. Mode of action uncertain. Used in treatment of arthritis. May cause severe diarrhoea. Other adverse effects include gastro-intestinal bleeding, exacerbation of asthma, haemolytic anaemia, and bone marrow depression. May enhance action of oral anticoagulants (e.g., WARFARIN).

Mefloquine. Antimalarial effective in treatment and prevention of infections resistant to CHLOROQUINE and other antimalarials. Like CHLOROQUINE it is a derivative of QUININE but has longer actions requiring only weekly dosage for prophylaxis. May cause dizziness, gastro-intestinal disturbances, rashes and severe neuropsychiatric reactions. May increase the risk of convulsions in epileptic patients. Also a risk of fatal arrhythmias if given together with HALOFANTRINE.

Mefruside. Diuretic essentially similar to BENDROFLUAZIDE.

Megestrol. Sex hormone, with actions and effects similar to PROGESTERONE. Used to suppress OESTROGEN-dependent tumours of the breast and the uterus by interfering with uptake of oestrogen into the tumour. Adverse effects include weight gain, nausea, skin rashes, hair loss, deep venous thromboses in the legs.

Meloxicam. Non-steroidal anti-inflammatory analgesic used in treatment of arthritis and ankylosing spondylitis. Specifically inhibits cyclo-oxygenase 2 (COX-2) rather than COX-1 and thus should be less likely to cause adverse effects on gastric mucosa (bleeding) and kidneys. May cause gastro-intestinal disturbance, skin reactions, CNS or cardiovascular effects and blood dyscrasias.

Melphalan. Cytotoxic drug used in myelomatosis. Actions and adverse effects similar to CHLORAMBUCIL.

Menadiol. Orally active form of VITAMIN K.

Menaphthone. *See* VITAMIN K.

Menotrophin. Preparation of follicle-stimulating hormone, derived from human post-menopausal urine, which also possesses some luteinizing hormone activity. Used to stimulate ovulation.

Menthol. Used as inhalation, orally as pastilles for relief of respiratory symptoms, or topically on skin where it causes dilatation of blood vessels producing a sense of coldness and analgesia.

Mepenzolate. Anticholinergic, with actions and adverse effects similar to ATROPINE. Marked effect upon spasm of colon. Used to relieve pain, distension, and diarrhoea associated with gastro-intestinal disorders.

Mepivacaine. Local anaesthetic with actions, adverse effects, and uses similar to LIGNOCAINE but not used to treat abnormal heart rhythms.

Meprobamate. Minor tranquillizer (anxiolytic) with selective action on hypothalamus and spinal cord. Used in treatment of neuroses, alcoholism, and functional disorders, such as tension headache. May cause gastro-intestinal disorders, headache, dizziness with hypotension, lowered tolerance to alcohol, and withdrawal symptoms. Induces hepatic drug metabolism with danger of drug interactions. Coma with respiratory depression in overdosage. No antidote. Forced alkaline diuresis and haemodialysis may be effective.

Meptazinol. Analgesic with narcotic antagonist activity. Actions, uses and adverse effects similar to PENTAZOCINE, but central adverse effects and dependence appear to be less.

Mequitazine. Antihistamine with actions and adverse effects similar to PROMETHAZINE. Used in treatment of allergic conditions.

Mercaptopurine. Cytotoxic drug, inhibiting nucleoprotein synthesis, used in neoplastic disease, particularly leukaemia. Adverse effects include bone marrow depression.

Meropenem. Intravenous broad spectrum antibiotic with actions, uses and adverse effects similar to IMIPENEM. Unlike IMIPENEM it does not need the addition of CILASTATIN to prolong its action.

Mersalyl. Organic mercurial diuretic, now seldom used. Depresses active reabsorption of sodium and chloride by kidney tubules. Long-acting; must be administered by intramuscular injection. Danger of excessive loss of sodium and chloride. May cause gastro-intestinal disturbance, skin rashes, and, after prolonged use, kidney damage.

Mesalazine (5-Aminosalicylic acid). Active constituent of SULPHASALAZINE. Used in ulcerative colitis. Free of sulphonamide adverse effects. Both by mouth and as an enema.

Mescaline (m). A hallucinogenic alkaloid obtained from the Mexican cactus *Lophophora williamsii* (Aztec name, Peyote), usually taken by mouth. Actions and adverse effects said to be similar to LSD but milder. Mescaline is abused in USA but less commonly in Europe. Peyote has a long tradition of use by Indians of northern Mexico and southwestern United States as a hallucinogen and medicine. Tolerance may occur but not physical dependence. Overdose does not cause serious physiological effects. No accepted medical usage.

Mesna. Used to protect the bladder mucosa from the irritant effect upon it of CYCLOPHOSPHAMIDE and IFOSFAMIDE. Acts by combining with their toxic metabolite acrolein. Does not prevent their other toxic effects.

Mesterolone. Sex hormone, with actions, uses, and adverse effects similar to TESTOSTERONE.

Mestranol. Sex hormone, with actions, uses, and adverse effects similar to ESTRADIOL.

Metaraminol. Sympathomimetic agent with alpha- and beta-effects similar to ADRENALINE. Alpha-effects predominate and thus it has been used to raise blood pressure in hypotension after myocardial infarction. May cause headache, dizziness, nausea, vomiting, and tremor.

Metformin. Oral antidiabetic. Increases use of glucose by peripheral tissues. Used alone or in combination with sulphonylureas (e.g., CHLORPROPAMIDE) or INSULIN. Most useful in overweight subjects, where it suppresses appetite. May cause nausea, vomiting, and diarrhoea.

Methacholine. Parasympathomimetic drug, with muscarinic actions of ACETYLCHOLINE.

Methacycline. Antibacterial, with actions, uses, and adverse effects similar to TETRACYCLINE.

Methadone (c). Synthetic narcotic analgesic. Actions similar to MORPHINE, but less sedation, euphoria, and respiratory depression. Used in control of withdrawal symptoms from narcotic addiction and for relief of chronic pain in terminal disease. NALOXONE is a pure antagonist.

Methallenestril. Sex hormone, with actions, uses, and adverse effects similar to OESTRADIOL.

Methaqualone (c). Hypnotic/sedative. General depressant action on CNS. Used in treatment in insomnia. Frequently has 'hangover' effect. May also cause localized loss of sensation with numbness and tingling, as well as skin rashes and gastro-intestinal disturbance. Liable to abuse for so-called 'aphrodisiac' qualities and euphoriant effects. In overdose causes respiratory depression with increased muscle tone and increased reflexes. No antidote. Treatment is supportive.

Methenamine. rINN for HEXAMINE.

Methicillin. Antibiotic. Similar properties to CLOXACILLIN, but only active parenterally.

Methionine. Amino acid, essential constituent of diet. May be used as an antidote in severe poisoning due to PARACETAMOL where it is thought to prevent liver damage by reducing the concentration of a toxic metabolite. Given orally it causes few side effects, principally nausea. Must not be given more than ten hours after the overdose as it may then exacerbate liver damage.

Methocarbamol. Muscle relaxant used in treatment of painful muscle spasms. Mode of action uncertain. May cause nausea, dizziness, drowsiness, headache, blurred vision and allergic reactions. Contraindicated in patients with epilepsy or myasthenia gravis.

Methohexital. rINN for METHOHEXITONE.

Methohexitone. Ultra-short-acting barbiturate hypnotic. Used for induction of anaesthesia. Actions and adverse effects similar to THIOPENTONE SODIUM.

Methoserpidine. Antihypertensive. Actions, uses, and adverse effects similar to RESERPINE.

Methotrexate. Cytotoxic drug, antagonizing folic acid, used in neoplastic disease, particularly leukaemia. Adverse effects include alopecia, stomatitis, liver toxicity, folate-deficient anaemia, and bone marrow depression.

Methotrimeprazine. Antipsychotic, with actions, uses, and adverse effects similar to CHLORPROMAZINE.

Methoxamine. Sympathomimetic. Stimulates alpha-adrenoceptors to cause constriction of blood vessels and rise in blood pressure. Used to reverse hypotension during anaesthesia. May cause pronounced slowing of heart rate and excessive rise in blood pressure.

Methoxydesethylamphetamine. *See* MDEA.

Methoxydesmethylamphetamine. *See* MDA.

5-Methoxypsoralen. Sun screen. Used topically to filter out harmful sun rays. May cause photosensitivity and has been suspected of increasing the incidence of skin cancer.

Methylcellulose. Indigestible plant residue used as a lubricating agent in pharmaceutical preparations and as a purgative. Adsorbs water, increases faecal bulk and thus promotes bowel movements. Slow action (0.5–3 days). No important systemic effects.

Methylcysteine. Mucolytic, with actions, uses, and adverse effects similar to ACETYLCYSTEINE. Used orally as well as by aerosol inhalation.

Methyldopa. Antihypertensive. Reduces sympathetic tone by central and peripheral mechanisms. Adverse effects include sedation, depression, nasal stuffiness, fluid retention, impotence, and haemolytic anaemia.

Methylenedioxymethamphetamine. *See* MDMA.

Methylephedrine. Sympathomimetic agent, with actions, uses, and adverse effects similar to EPHEDRINE.

Methyl nicotinate. Vasodilator/rubefacient used in ointments and creams for topical application at sites of muscle pains in rheumatic conditions (e.g fibrositis, muscular rheumatism).

Methylphenobarbital. rINN for METHYLPHENOBARBITONE.

Methylphenobarbitone (c). Anticonvulsant/sedative essentially similar to PHENOBARBITONE.

Methylprednisolone. CORTICOSTEROID with actions, uses, and adverse effects similar to PREDNISONE.

Methyl salicylate. Rubefacient used for relief of musculo-skeletal pain. Has similar actions and adverse effects to ACETYLSALICYLIC ACID but not used systemically.

Methyltestosterone. Sex hormone, with actions, uses and adverse effects similar to TESTOSTERONE.

Methysergide. Serotonin antagonist used in preventive treatment for severe migraine. May cause nausea, abdominal cramp, dizziness, and psychiatric disturbance. Prolonged use may cause retroperitoneal fibrosis resulting in impairment of renal function.

Metipranolol. Beta-adrenoceptor blocking drug with actions and adverse effects similar to PROPRANOLOL, but used only as eyedrops for glaucoma. *See also* TIMOLOL.

Metirosine. Antihypertensive. Enzyme inhibitor which blocks the syntheses of catecholamines by the adrenal gland. Used to control hypertension caused by the adrenal tumour phaeochromocytoma where the raised blood pressure is caused by excess production of catecholamines. Adverse effects include sedation, diarrhoea, and hypersensitivity.

Metoclopramide. Antiemetic with dopamine antagonist actions in brain and peripheral effects on gastro-intestinal tract where it stimulates motility to improve gastric emptying and intestinal transit. May cause drowsiness and involuntary movements. Used to treat nausea and vomiting from most causes and as an adjunct to X-ray examination of the gut.

Metolazone. Diuretic essentially similar to BENDROFLUAZIDE.

Metoprolol. Beta-adrenoceptor blocking drug, with limited cardioselectivity. Uses, side effects, etc. as for PROPRANOLOL.

Metriphonate. Organophosphorus cholinesterase inhibitor, used as an anti-infective in treatment of schistosomiasis. Active only against S. *haematobium.* May cause unwanted cholinergic symptoms as from ACETYLCHOLINE.

Metronidazole. Antimicrobial. Effective against trichomonas, Vincent' s organisms, anaerobic bacteria, giardiasis, and amoebiasis. Adverse effects include nausea, metallic taste in mouth, hypersensitivity reactions, DISULFIRAM-like reaction with alcohol.

Metyrapone. Inhibits enzyme responsible for synthesis of adrenocorticosteroids. Used in tests of pituitary gland function. May cause gastro-intestinal disturbance and dizziness.

Mexenone. Absorbs ultraviolet light and protects skin from sunburn.

Mexiletine. Cardiac antiarrhythmic agent similar to LIGNOCAINE, but also effective when given by mouth. May cause nausea, vomiting, drowsiness, tremors, convulsions, hypotension, and bradycardia.

Mianserin. Antidepressant, with uses similar to IMIPRAMINE, but without its peripheral autonomic adverse effects. Produces sedation and a fall in white blood cell count in some patients.

Mibefradil. Calcium antagonist acting upon the T-type (transient) calcium channels rather than the L (long-lasting) calcium channels. Causes reduced cardiac contraction and conductivity plus vasodilatation. Used in treatment of high blood pressure and prevention of angina. May cause excessive slowing of the heart with consequent arrhythmias and cardiac failure.

Miconazole. Antifungal agent used topically for skin infections.

Midazolam. Intravenous benzodiazepine anxiolytic/sedative, with short duration of action. Used for induction of anaesthesia before minor surgery. Actions and adverse effects similar to DIAZEPAM.

Mifepristone. Progesterone antagonist used orally for termination of pregnancy up to 9 weeks gestation. May cause skin rashes, general malaise and gastro-intestinal disturbance. Used only in centres licensed under the abortion act. If abortion is not complete after 36–48 hours, treatment with GEMEPROST should be given. Surgical abortion may be used if drug treatment fails.

Milrinone. Phosphodiesterase enzyme inhibitor which reduces breakdown of cyclic AMP and thus prolongs its effects in contraction of cardiac and relaxation of vascular smooth muscle. Used to improve cardiac output in severe congestive cardiac failure. May cause hypotension, angina, cardiac arrhythmias and headache.

Mineral oil. *See* LIQUID PARAFFIN.

Minocycline. Antibacterial, with actions, uses, and adverse effects similar to TETRACYCLINE. May cause dizziness and vertigo.

Minoxidil. Vasodilator/antihypertensive. Reduces muscle tone in peripheral blood vessels. Fluid retention and tachycardia accompany this effect but can be controlled by using concomitant therapy with a diuretic (e.g., BENDROFLUAZIDE) and a beta-adrenoceptor blocker (e.g., PROPRANOLOL). Other adverse effects include increase hair growth and breast tenderness. Used mainly in severe hypertension when other drugs fail. It is also used topically to treat male-pattern baldness, but the effects appear limited and reverse when treatment is stopped.

Mirtazapine. Antidepressant which increases both noradrenergic and serotonergic nerve transmission in the brain. Does not show the unwanted anticholinergic activity of the tricyclic antidepressants e.g. AMITRIPTYLINE. May cause drowsiness, weight gain and peripheral oedema. Toxic effects in the liver and bone marrow have been described.

Misoprostol. Synthetic analogue of endogenously produced prostaglandin PGE_1 that promotes the healing of duodenal and gastric ulcers and ulcers induced by non-steroid anti-inflammatory drugs. It also protects the gastric mucosa against initial damage. It inhibits production of gastric acid, stimulating bicarbonate and mucus secretion and maintaining mucosal blood flow. May cause diarrhoea, abnormal vaginal bleeding and abortion.

Mithramycin. Cytotoxic antibiotic. No longer used to treat cancer itself, but may be used as emergency therapy to reduce hypercalcaemia due to malignant disease. More effective than chelating agents such as TRI-SODIUM EDETATE, but causes suppression of bone marrow and cannot be used for more than a few days.

Mitomycin. Cytotoxic antibiotic. Used to treat upper gastro-intestinal and breast cancers. Causes delayed effects on the bone marrow, lung fibrosis, and renal damage. Used at six-week intervals to reduce these effects.

Mitoxantrone. rINN for MITOZANTRONE.

Mitozantrone. Cytotoxic drug, with actions against resting-phase tumour, as well as those undergoing DNA synthesis. May thus be effective in both slow and rapid growing tumours. Used in advanced breast cancer. May cause bone marrow suppression, hair loss, gastro-intestinal disturbances, heart failure and impaired liver function.

Mivacurium. Skeletal muscle relaxant with actions similar to TUBOCURARINE, but a shorter duration of action.

Mizolastine. Non-sedating antihistamine with actions and uses similar to TERFENADINE. Although minor ECG changes are seen there have been no reports of cardiac arrhythmias.

Moclobemide. Antidepressant. Acts by selective inhibition of monoamine oxidase enzyme type A (MAO-A) in the brain. Increases brain monoamines by reducing their enzymic breakdown. Acts more rapidly than earlier MAOIs such as PHENELZINE, and causes fewer adverse effects. May cause sleep disturbance, agitation, nausea and headache. May interact with tricyclic and tetracyclic antidepressants and with TRAZODONE.

Modafinil. Non-AMPHETAMINE CNS stimulant used in the treatment of the chronic sleep disorder narcolepsy. Acts by blocking the release of the inhibitory neurotransmitter GABA. Does not affect DOPAMINE release and thus hyperkinesia is not a problem. The incidence of euphoria is low and consequently abuse is unlikely. May cause headache and unwanted CNS excitation e.g. aggression or insomnia.

Moexipril. Pro-drug for moexiprilat a potent inhibitor of angiotensin converting enzyme, with actions similar to CAPTOPRIL. Used alone or in combination therapy for hypertension. Adverse effects include cough, headache, dizziness, fatigue, flushing and rash.

Molgramostim. Human growth factor made by recombinant DNA technology with actions and uses similar to FILGRASTIM.

Mometasone. Corticosteroid nasal spray for use in symptomatic relief and prevention of hayfever. Actions, uses and adverse effects similar to intranasal BECLOMETHASONE.

Mometasone. Potent synthetic CORTICOSTEROID similar to DEXAMETHASONE.

Monosulfiram. Parasiticide used topically for treatment of fleas, lice, ticks and mites. May cause skin rashes. Related to DISULFIRAM and may have similar effects if ingested.

Montelukast. Oral leukotriene receptor antagonist. Blocks part of the inflammatory process associated with an asthma attack and thus helps to reduce swelling/constriction of the airways. Used as an add-on therapy in the long term management of asthma when treatment with inhaled corticosteroids and beta-adrenoceptor stimulants is inadequate. May cause headache and abdominal pain.

Moracizine. Antiarrhythmic with similarities to DISOPYRAMIDE, used to suppress abnormal ventricular rhythms. Has a relatively long duration of action due to active metabolites. May cause dizziness, arrhythmias, gastro-intestinal disturbance, muscle pain and blurred vision.

Morphine (c). Poppy derivative. Centrally acting narcotic analgesic used for relief of severe pain. Other potentially useful effects include euphoria and cough suppression. Adverse effects include respiratory depression, nausea, vomiting, constipation, hypotension, physical dependence, and ('addiction') abuse. Coma with danger of death in overdosage. NALOXONE is a specific antagonist.

Moxisylyte. rINN for THYMOXAMINE.

Moxonidine. Antihypertensive acts on imidazoline sub-type 1 receptors to the brain medulla. Used alone or in combination therapy to reduce mild to moderate blood pressure. May cause dry mouth, headache, nausea and insomnia.

Mupirocin. Antibiotic, previously known as pseudomonic acid. Used as an ointment to treat bacterial skin infections. Inactive orally.

Mustine hydrochloride (Nitrogen mustard). Cytotoxic drug used in neoplastic disease. Adverse effects include nausea, vomiting, and bone marrow depression.

Mycophenolate. Immunosupressant, prodrug, metabolised to mycophenolic acid which inhibits lymphocyte production. Used to prevent rejection of kidney transplants. May cause gastro-intestinal upsets, bone marrow suppression, CNS disturbance and increased susceptibility to infection.

N

Nabilone. Derivative of cannabis, with antiemetic and anxiolytic properties. Acts on opiate receptors in the brain to block transmission of vomiting impulses. Used to suppress nausea and vomiting from cytotoxic drugs. Adverse effects include drowsiness, postural hypotension, headaches, tremors, psychosis, and abdominal cramps.

Nabumetone. Non-steroid anti-inflammatory/analgesic, used in osteoarthritis and rheumatoid arthritis. The drug itself is a relatively weak inhibitor of prostaglandin synthesis, but it is metabolized in the liver to a more active compound. May thus cause less gastro-intestinal irritation than some other drugs in this class such as INDOMETHACIN, but is still contraindicated if there is a history of peptic ulceration. May cause diarrhoea, other gastro-intestinal symptoms, headache, dizziness, rashes and sedation.

Nadolol. Beta-adrenoceptor blocking drug. Uses and adverse effects as for PROPRANOLOL.

Nafarelin. Synthetic analogue of gonadotrophin-releasing hormone. Used by nasal spray in the treatment of endometriosis. May cause hot flushes, changes in libido, headaches and muscle pains.

Naftidrofuryl. Peripheral vasodilator said to improve cellular metabolism and to relax muscle cells in blood vessel walls. Recommended for treatment of reduced peripheral blood circulation and dementia caused by reduced blood flow. May cause headache, insomnia, and gastro-intestinal disturbance.

Nalbuphine. Narcotic analgesic, with agonist and antagonist properties. Uses and adverse effects similar to PENTAZOCINE.

Nalidixic acid. Urinary antiseptic to which resistance readily occurs. May cause gastro-intestinal symptoms and allergic reactions. May exacerbate epilepsy and respiratory depression.

Nalorphine. Narcotic antagonist. Reverses effects of MORPHINE and other narcotic analgesics but less specific than NALOXONE and has some narcotic activity of its own. Used for reversal of narcotic effects but not when due to PENTAZOCINE. May cause hallucinations and thought disturbances. In 'addicts', causes severe withdrawal symptoms.

Naloxone. Narcotic antagonist. A true antidote to MORPHINE and other narcotic analgesics. Has no narcotic activity in its own right. Used for reversal of narcotic effects from any narcotic drug especially respiratory depression. Danger of severe withdrawal symptoms if given to those physically dependent ('addicted') on narcotics.

Naltrexone. Narcotic antagonist which acts as an antidote to MORPHINE and other narcotic analgesics, with virtually no narcotic activity of its own. Unlike NALOXONE can be given orally and has a long duration of action. Used to promote opioid abstinence in patients who were formerly drug-dependent. May cause drowsiness, anxiety, loss of appetite, nausea, vomiting, diarrhoea or constipation, muscle and joint pains.

Nandrolone. Sex hormone, with actions and adverse effects similar to TESTOS-

TERONE, but anabolic effects greater than androgenic effects. Used in treatment of debilitating illness and carcinoma of the breast. Injection only; not active by mouth.

Naphazoline. Sympathomimetic agent with marked alpha-adrenergic activity. Used topically on nasal mucosa where its vasoconstrictor effect leads to reduced secretion and mucosal swelling (e.g., in allergic rhinitis). Prolonged use may lead to rebound nasal congestion and secretion. Not used systemically but oral overdosage would cause depression of nervous system and coma.

Naproxen. Anti-inflammatory/analgesic, with actions, uses, and adverse effects similar to IBUPROFEN.

Naratriptan. Oral 5-HYDROXYTRYPTAMINE agonist with actions and adverse effects similar to SUMATRIPTAN. Used in treatment of acute migraine attacks.

Nedocromil. Preventive treatment for asthma and bronchitis with reversible obstruction of the airways. Acts like SODIUM CROMOGLYCATE by blocking allergic mechanisms. Administered by aerosol. May cause headache and nausea. Also used topically as eye drops for allergic conjunctivitis.

Nefazodone. Antidepressant with actions, uses and adverse effects similar to FLUOXETINE. May be particularly beneficial in cases with anxiety or insomnia.

Nefopam. Centrally acting analgesic; mode of action unknown, but not related to the narcotics. Used for acute and chronic pain. Adverse effects include gastrointestinal upsets, palpitations, and CNS stimulation with nervousness, insomnia, headache, blurred vision, and sweating. Drowsiness is sometimes seen, but respiratory depression and habituation do not occur. Contraindicated in patients with epilepsy, glaucoma, or urinary retention.

Nelfinavir. Antiviral agent used in combined therapy for HIV. May cause gastrointestinal disturbance, rash and possibly altered liver function.

Neomycin. Bactericidal aminoglycoside antibiotic with spectrum similar to STREPTOMYCIN, but more active against *Stalphylococcus* and *Proteus.* Not used systemically because of risk of ototoxicity and nephrotoxicity. Used topically and orally for bowel sterilization and in liver failure. May cause malabsorption if given for long period. Potentiates neuromuscular blockade.

Neostigmine (Prostigmine). Anticholinesterase with actions similar to PHYSOSTIGMINE.

Netilmicin. Aminoglycoside antibiotic, with actions, uses, and adverse effects similar to GENTAMICIN.

Nevirapine. Antiviral agent used in combined therapy for HIV. May cause gastrointestinal disturbance, rash and possibly altered liver function.

Niacinamide. Vitamin: *see* NICOTINIC ACID.

Nialamide. Antidepressant/monoamine oxidase inhibitor with actions, uses, and adverse effects similar to PHENELZINE.

Nicardipine. Anti-anginal, antihypertensive with actions, uses and adverse effects similar to NIFEDIPINE.

Niclosamide. Used in treatment of tapeworms. Adverse effects are uncommon as it is not absorbed from the intestinal tract.

Nicofuranose. *See* TETRANICOTINOYLFRUCTOSE.

Nicorandil. Potassium channel blocker. Acts on muscle cells in coronary arteries and veins to cause dilation and improved blood flow. Used to prevent and treat angina. May cause headaches, flushing and fall in blood pressure.

Nicotinamide. The active form of Niacin (Vitamin B_3) used in multivitamin preparations. Also posessses anti-inflammatory properties and is used topically in the treatment of acne. When used topically may cause dry itchy skin.

Nicotine. Plant derivative from the tobacco plant *(Nicotiana* spp). Nicotine is the addictive component in tobacco smoke. Addiction is physiological and psychological and many smokers find it difficult to stop, even when they have illnesses which are made worse by smoking. Nicotine may be administered during the withdrawal period in the form of transdermal patches or chewing gum.

Nicotinic acid (Vitamin B_7). Vitamin. Deficiency causes pellagra, with dermatitis, diarrhoea, and dementia. Has direct relaxant effect on muscle in peripheral blood vessels and has been used to treat reduced peripheral circulation. Large doses may cause flushing and gastro-intestinal symptoms.

Nicotinyl tartrate. Peripheral vasodilator acting directly on muscle in blood vessels. Used for treatment of impaired peripheral blood circulation including chilblains and Raynaud's syndrome. May cause flushing, tachycardia, shivering, gastro-intestinal symptoms, and fall in blood pressure.

Nicoumalone. Anticoagulant, with actions, interactions, and adverse effects similar to WARFARIN.

Nifedipine. Antianginal/antihypertensive vasodilator. Acts by blocking influx of calcium ions into vascular smooth muscle thus reducing peripheral vascular resistance. Adverse effects include flushing, headache, and lethargy. In overdosage, causes bradycardia and hypotension, which may be treated by ATROPINE, DOPAMINE, and CALCIUM GLUCONATE.

Nikethamide. Respiratory stimulant acting directly on brain respiratory centres. Seldom useful except in respiratory depression due to severe chronic bronchitis. Not used in treatment of respiratory depression due to drug overdosage. May cause sweating, nausea, vomiting, convulsions, and depression of the nervous system.

Nimodipine. Vasodilator used after subarachnoid haemorrhage to reverse spasms of the arteries which would cause ischaemia of the brain tissues. Reduces the contraction of vascular smooth muscle by blocking influx of calcium ions, similar in action to NIFEDIPINE.

Nimorazole. Antiprotozoal used to treat certain gastro-intestinal and vaginal infections (e.g., giardiasis, trichomoniasis). Contraindicated in neurological disease. Causes nausea if alcohol taken during treatment.

Niridazole. Used in treatment of infections due to the guinea worm *(Dracunculus medinensis).* May cause gastro-intestinal symptoms, headache, and drowsiness. Rare effects include confusion, convulsions, and allergic reactions.

Nisoldipine. Calcium antagonist with actions and adverse effects similar to AMLODIPINE. Used to treat hypertension and angina.

Nitrazepam (m). Benzodiazepine tranquillizer/hypnotic. Depressant action on CNS. Used in treatment of insomnia. May cause dizziness, unsteadiness, and slurred speech. In overdosage, respiratory depression much less severe than with barbiturates. No antidote; supportive treatment only. May cause dependence, even in therapeutic doses.

Nitrofurantoin. Urinary antiseptic, producing yellow fluorescence in urine. Adverse effects include hypersensitivity reactions, nausea, vomiting, and neuropathy, haemolytic anaemia in G6PD-deficient subjects.

Nitrogen mustard. *See* MUSTINE HYDROCHLORIDE.

Nitrophenol. Has antifungal activity. Used topically for fungal infections of the skin.

Nitrous oxide. Inhalational anaesthetic. Weak anaesthetic, but strong analgesic. Usually given with at least 30 percent oxygen (e.g., in dental and obstetric practice for light anaesthesia or for induction only in major surgery).

Nizatidine. Gastric histamine receptor blocker, with actions and uses similar to CIMETIDINE. May cause headache, tiredness, muscle pains, pharyngitis, cough, and sweating.

Nomifensine. Antidepressant, with actions, uses, and adverse effects similar to IMIPRAMINE. Recently withdrawn due to increasing reports of adverse effects, including haemolytic anaemia.

Nonoxynol. Nonionic surfactant used as spermicidal cream.

Nonylic acid. Rubefacient used topically for musculo-skeletal pain.

Noradrenaline. Sympathomimetic amine, predominantly alpha-adrenoceptor agonist. Produces general vasoconstriction with rise of blood pressure. Toxicity includes hypertension, cerebral haemorrhage, and pulmonary oedema.

Norepinephrine. rINN for NORADRENALINE.

Norethandrolone. Sex hormone with actions similar to TESTOSTERONE, but anabolic effects greater than androgenic effects. Active by mouth or by injection. Used to treat debilitating conditions and carcinoma of the breast. Used with caution if liver function is impaired.

Norethisterone. Sex hormone, with actions and adverse effects of PROGESTERONE. Used for contraception and treatment of uterine bleeding.

Norethynodrel. Sex hormone, with actions and adverse effects similar to PROGESTERONE. Used for contraception and treatment of uterine bleeding.

Norfloxacin. Broad spectrum antibiotic for urinary tract infections, with actions and adverse effects similar to CIPROFLOXACIN, but not available for intravenous use. Adverse effects include photosensitivity, hypersensitivity, pancreatitis, hepatitis, haemolytic anaemia, paraesthesia and confusion. Also used topically as eye drops.

Norgestimate. Synthetic progestogen used as an oral contraceptive, combined with an oestrogen. Adverse effects similar to other progestogens. Experimental studies suggest that it may have a beneficial effect on plasma lipids. Any benefit in reducing cardiovascular disease will only be revealed by long-term epidemiological studies.

Norgestrel. Sex hormone, with actions and adverse effects similar to PROGESTERONE. Used for oral contraception and subdermal long-term depot contraception.

Nortriptyline. Antidepressant, with actions, uses, and adverse effects similar to IMIPRAMINE.

Noscapine. Cough suppressant, with actions and adverse effects similar to PHOLCODINE.

Novobiocin. Antibiotic used for infections by PENICILLIN-resistant staphylococci. Adverse effects include hypersensitivity reactions with urticarial rashes and kernicterus in the neonate.

Noxythiolin. Anti-infective with antibacterial and antifungal activity. Used topically for prevention or treatment of infections in bladder or other body cavities (e.g., after bladder operations).

Nystatin. Antibiotic used in treatment of *Candida* infections of skin and mucous membranes, particularly mouth, alimentary tract, and vagina.

O

Octocog alfa. Blood clotting factor that is deficient in haemophilia and Von Willbrand's disease. Used intravenously to stop episodes of uncontrollable bleeding.

Octoxynol. Nonionic surfactant. Used as spermicidal cream.

Octreotide. A synthetic analogue of somatostatin which reduces blood levels of growth hormone and THYROTROPHIN and inhibits INSULIN and GLUCAGON release. Used to relieve the symptoms of gastro-pancreatic endocrine tumours. May cause pain at injection and gastro-intestinal disturbance.

Oestradiol. Naturally occurring sex hormone (OESTROGEN). Controls development and function of female sex organs, working in conjunction with PROGESTERONE. Could be used for menstrual disorders, oestrogen deficiency, oral contraception, and suppression of certain neoplastic disease, but mainly superseded by related compounds. Also used for prevention of osteoporosis. May cause withdrawal bleeding, breast development in the male, salt and water retention, nausea and vomiting, stimulation of tumours and arterial and venous thrombosis. Use avoided in patients with known risks of these effects.

Oestriol. Sex hormone (OESTROGEN) similar to OESTRADIOL, but more active by mouth. Used mainly for menopausal disorders.

Oestrogen. Sex hormone: *see* OESTRADIOL, OESTRIOL and OESTRONE.

Oestrone. Sex hormone (OESTROGEN) similar to OESTRADIOL. Used mainly for menopausal disorders.

Ofloxacin. Synthetic antibacterial related to NALIDIXIC ACID, used to treat infections of lower respiratory tract, urinary tract, genital tract and eye. Adverse effects include dizziness, visual disturbances, gastro-intestinal disturbances, tendon damage and allergic reactions.

Olanzapine. Antipsychotic with actions similar to CLOZAPINE but thought to be free of its adverse effects on the bone marrow. Used to treat schizophrenia. May cause drowsiness, weight gain and dizziness.

Oleandomycin. Antibiotic, with similar actions and adverse effects to ERYTHROMYCIN.

Olsalazine. Used to treat and prevent relapse of ulcerative colitis. Consists of two joined molecules of MESALAZINE, the active compound released when SULPHASALAZINE is metabolized. This breakdown of the molecule occurs in the colon where it is required. Thought to act by inhibiting prostaglandin synthesis. May cause diarrhoea, abdominal cramps, headache, nausea, dyspepsia, arthralgia and rashes.

Omeprazole. For benign peptic ulcers and oesophageal reflux. Reduces gastric acid secretion by acting directly on its production. Adverse effects include headache, nausea, and rashes.

Ondansetron. Anti-emetic with actions on 5-HYDROXYTRYPTAMINE receptors in the brain and gastro-intestinal tract, used to treat vomiting induced by anti-cancer drugs and radiotherapy and occurring after surgery. Adverse effects include constipation, headache and rarely, hypersensitivity reactions.

Opium tincture (c). Mixture of poppy alkaloids: *see* MORPHINE.

Orciprenaline. Beta-adrenoceptor agonist used in bronchial asthma. Adverse effects include tachycardia, arrhythmias, and tremor.

Orphenadrine. Parasympatholytic/antihistamine. Used as antispasmodic in treatment of parkinsonism. Actions, adverse effect, etc. as for BENZHEXOL.

Ouabain. Plant derivative with effects on the heart similar to those of DIGOXIN, but only reliably active when given by injection when the onset of action is more rapid than for digoxin.

Oxamniquine. Anti-infective for treatment of schistosomiasis due to *S. mansoni.* Adverse effects include transient fever and dizziness.

Oxatomide. Antihistamine that blocks histamine H_1 receptors and release of allergic mediators from mast cells. Used in treatment of allergies (e.g., hay fever, urticaria) but not asthma. Adverse effects similar to PROMETHAZINE (i.e. drowsiness, potentiation of alcohol). In high doses, causes reversible weight gain.

Oxazepam. Benzodiazepine anxiolytic similar to DIAZEPAM.

Ox bile extract. Recommended for treatment of biliary deficiency. Probably of little use, except that it increases bowel activity and helps to relieve constipation.

Oxetacaine. rINN for OXETHAZAINE.

Oxethazaine. Surface-active local anaesthetic. Added to some antacid mixtures with intention of adding an analgesic effect. Actions and adverse effects similar to LIGNOCAINE.

Oxitropium. Anticholinergic with a local effect on the lungs used by inhalation as a bronchodilator in chronic asthma and chronic obstructive lung disease. May cause anticholinergic side effects similar to those of ATROPINE SULPHATE, such as dry mouth, blurred vision and urinary retention. Should not be used in patients with glaucoma or prostatic hypertrophy.

Oxolinic acid. Urinary antiseptic for treatment of urine infections. May cause gastro-intestinal symptoms and CNS stimulation. Contraindicated in epilepsy.

Oxpentifylline. *See* OXYPENTIFYLLINE.

Oxprenolol. Beta-adrenoceptor blocking drug with partial agonist activity (intrinsic sympathomimetic activity). Uses, side effects, etc. as for PROPRANOLOL.

Oxybuprocaine. Local anaesthetic for topical use. Similar to AMETHOCAINE, but less likely to cause irritation.

Oxybutynin. Anticholinergic with antispasmodic activity used to relax bladder in treatment of urinary frequency and incontinence, and nocturnal enuresis in children. Side effects similar to those of ATROPINE SULPHATE.

Oxymetazoline. Sympathomimetic with marked alpha-adrenergic effects. Used topically on nasal mucosa as treatment for nasal congestion. Actions and adverse effects similar to NAPHAZOLINE.

Oxymetholone. Sex hormone, with similar actions, uses, and adverse effects to TESTOSTERONE.

Oxypentifylline. Vasodilator used in treatment of peripheral vascular disease (e.g., intermittent claudication, Raynaud's syndrome). May reduce blood pressure, lower blood glucose, or cause gastro-intestinal symptoms. May cause nausea, dizziness, flushing, and hypotension. Caution needed if given with antihypertensives or insulin as it may increase their effects.

Oxypertine. Tranquillizer used in treatment of schizophrenia, other psychoses and anxiety neuroses. May cause drowsiness (high doses) or hyperactivity (low doses). Gastro-intestinal disturbances, hypotension, and involuntary movements less frequent than with the phenothiazines. Coma with respiratory depression in overdosage. No antidote; supportive treatment only.

Oxyphenbutazone. Anti-inflammatory/analgesic essentially similar to PHENYLBUTAZONE of which it is a metabolite. Now discontinued orally because of high incidence of adverse reactions. Still used topically in eye.

Oxyphenisatin. Laxative used in preparative enemas before radiology, endoscopy, or surgery.

Oxyquinoline. Has antibacterial, antifungal, deodorant, and keratolytic properties. Used topically on skin or in vagina for minor infections and acne. Sensitivity rashes may occur.

Oxytetracycline. Bacteriostatic antibiotic, with actions, adverse effects, and interactions similar to TETRACYCLINE.

Oxytocin. Hormone from the posterior pituitary gland. Causes contraction of uterus. Used for induction of labour. May cause fluid retention and uterine rupture with danger to foetus. Contraindicated in toxaemia of pregnancy, placental abnormalities, or foetal distress.

P

Paclitaxel. Cytotoxic agent used in treatment of patients with advanced ovarian cancer resistant to CISPLATIN-based chemotherapy and in metastatic breast cancer resistant to anthracycline therapy. May cause bone marrow suppression, peripheral neuropathy, arthralgia and myalgia.

Pamidronate. Reduces serum calcium in tumour induced hypercalcaemia but has a slow onset of action so is not suitable for initial treatment of severe hypercalcaemia. Inhibits bone resorption, so is used to treat Paget's disease, osteolytic lesions and bone pain associated with multiple myeloma and breast cancer. Adverse effects include transient reduction in lymphocyte count, fever and reduced urine output.

Pancreatic enzymes. Extracts of animal pancreas. Used to aid digestion of starch, fats, and protein when there is pancreatic deficiency. May cause sore mouth and sensitivity reactions with sneezing, watery eyes or skin rashes. Has been associated with fibrosis of the colon in children under 15 years.

Pancreatin. *See* PANCREATIC ENZYMES.

Pancuronium. Muscle relaxant with actions and uses similar to TUBOCURARINE.

Panthenol. *See* PANTOTHENIC ACID.

Pantoprazole. For benign peptic ulcers and oesophageal reflux. Reduces gastric acid secretion by acting directly on its production. Adverse effects include headaches, nausea and rashes.

Pantothenic acid. Considered a vitamin, but no proven deficiency disease in man. No accepted therapeutic role, but included in some vitamin mixtures.

Papaveretum (c). Mixture of poppy derivatives; 50 per cent is MORPHINE, to which it is similar in all respects.

Papaverine. Muscle relaxant, with action on involuntary muscle. Used in bronchodilator aerosol mixtures and as relaxant in mixtures for gastro-intestinal spasm. Also used by direct injection into the penis to produce erection in erectile impotence. Low toxicity except intravenously when it may cause cardiac arrhythmias.

***para*-Aminobenzoic acid.** Nutrient. Essential metabolite for certain bacteria. Sometimes included in vitamin mixtures but there is no evidence of a deficiency disease in man. Large doses may cause nausea, skin rashes, and hypoglycaemia.

***para*-Aminosalicylic acid** (PAS). Synthetic anti-tuberculous agent, usually given as the sodium salt. Adverse effects include hypersensitivity reactions, nausea, vomiting, goitre, hypothyroidism, and hepatitis.

Paracetamol (Acetaminophen–USA). Analgesic/ antipyretic. Inhibits synthesis of prostaglandins in the brain but, unlike ACETYLSALICYLIC ACID, does not have this action in the periphery and therefore has no anti-inflammatory effect. Relieves mild pain but not inflammation. Overdosage may cause potentially fatal liver damage. ACETYLCYSTEINE and METHIONINE are antidotes.

Paradichlorobenzene. Insecticide included in some ear drops. May irritate the skin. Inhalation or ingestion may cause drowsiness.

Paraldehyde. Anticonvulsant/hypnotic/sedative. Used in status epilepticus or disturbed patients. Administered by intramuscular injection. Dissolves plastic syringes: glass must be used. Irritant at injection site. Exhaled in breath producing unpleasant odour.

Parathyroid hormone. Extract from parathyroid glands. Increases plasma calcium by mobilizing calcium from bone, reducing urine calcium excretion, and increasing its absorption from the gastro-intestinal tract. Active only by injection. Used to treat low plasma calcium (tetany). May cause abnormally high plasma calcium with weakness, lethargy, and coma.

Paroxetine. Antidepressant. Actions similar to FLUVOXAMINE. Adverse effects include nausea, somnolence, sweating, tremor, asthenia, dry mouth, insomnia, and sexual dysfunction.

PAS. *See para*-AMINOSALICYLIC ACID.

Pectin. Emulsifying agent, used in preparation of pharmaceutical and cosmetic products.

Pemoline (c). CNS stimulant with action intermediate between CAFFEINE and AMPHETAMINE. Used as treatment for lethargy. May cause insomnia, anxiety, and rapid heart rate.

Penamecillin. Similar to PHENOXYMETHYLPENICILLIN.

Penciclovir. Topical antiviral cream for treatment of cold sores (herpes labialis). Actions similar to ACICLOVIR. May cause localised burning or stinging.

Penicillamine. Chelating agent. Binds certain toxic metals (e.g., copper) and increases their excretion. Used in treatment of metal poisoning and rheumatoid arthritis (where its mechanism of action is uncertain). May cause headache, fever, loss of taste, gastro-intestinal symptoms, kidney damage, and bone marrow depression.

Penicillins. Group of bactericidal antibiotics that act by inhibiting bacterial cell wall synthesis. Hypersensitivity cross-reactions occur to all.

Penicillin V. *See* PHENOXYMETHYLPENICILLIN.

Pentaerithrityl. rINN for PENTAERYTHRITOL.

Pentaerythritol tetranitrate. Vasodilator with longer, but milder, action than GLYCERYL TRINITRATE whose adverse effects it shares. Used to prevent angina attacks.

Pentagastrin. Synthetic gastro-intestinal hormone. Stimulates secretion of gastric acid, pepsin and pancreatic enzymes. Used by injection as test of gastric and pancreatic function. May cause nausea, flushing, dizziness, and fall in blood pressure.

Pentamidine. Antiprotozoal used in treatment of protozoal infections including leishmaniasis and *Pneumocystis carnii.* The latter is common in AIDs and HIV positive individuals for whom treatment and prophylaxis may be given as an inhaled (nebulized) spray. Adverse effects include hypotension, nausea, and vomiting.

Pentazocine (c). Narcotic analgesic more potent than CODEINE, but less potent than MORPHINE. Dependence and addiction less common than with MORPHINE. Some activity as a narcotic antagonist like NALOXONE. May cause bad dreams, hallucinations, withdrawal symptoms, also nausea, vomiting, dizziness, and drowsiness. Constipation, and rarely respiratory depression may occur after injections. NALOXONE but not NALORPHINE nor LEVALLORPHAN may be used as anta-gonists.

Pentostatin. Inhibits intracellular enzymes leading to arrest of cell division in 'hairy cell' leukaemia. Adverse effects include rash, bone marrow suppression, heart failure and general malaise.

Pentoxifylline. rINN for OXPENTIFYLLINE.

Peppermint oil. Essential oil used to relieve gastric and intestinal flatulence and colic (e.g., irritable bowel syndrome). Adverse effects include heartburn, bradycardia, muscle tremor, anxiety and allergic reactions to its menthol content.

Pepsin. Enzyme found in normal gastric juice. Controls breakdown of proteins. May be given to improve digestion when there is deficiency of pepsin secretion.

Pergolide. Dopamine agonist used in Parkinson's Disease as an adjunct to treatment with LEVODOPA when the latter treatment is seen to be losing it effectiveness. Adverse effects include nausea, indigestion, low blood pressure, confusion, hallucinations, dyskinesia, and impaired consciousness.

Pericyazine. Tranquillizer, with actions, uses, and adverse effects similar to CHLORPROMAZINE.

Perindopril. Antihypertensive with actions, uses and adverse effects similar to CAPTOPRIL. A prodrug, it is converted to Perindoprilat before exerting its effect.

Permethrin. Synthetic pyrethroid insecticide used to treat headlice. Has very low toxicity in man but the shampoo may cause irritation if it contacts the eyes.

Perphenazine. Phenothiazine tranquillizer similar to CHLORPROMAZINE, used in treatment of psychotic disorders, agitation, and confusion. Not recommended for children.

Pethidine (c). Synthetic narcotic analgesic essentially similar to MORPHINE. Used for relief of severe pain. May produce nausea, vomiting, dry mouth, euphoria, sedation, and respiratory depression. Coma with danger of death on overdosage. NALOXONE is a specific antagonist. Long-term use associated with tolerance, physical dependence, and ('addiction') abuse.

PGI_2. *See* EPOPROSTENOL.

Phenacetin. Analgesic/antipyretic, but not anti-inflammatory. Converted by the liver to PARACETAMOL which is the main active form. Available only in combined analgesic preparations. Does not cause gastric irritation but may cause haemolytic anaemia and methaemoglobinaemia. Has been associated with kidney damage (analgesic nephropathy) and is now withdrawn in the UK.

Phenazocine (c). Narcotic analgesic similar to MORPHINE, but causes less sedation, vomiting, and hypotension. More likely to depress respiration than morphine.

Phenazone. Analgesic/antipyretic. Local anaesthetic action when applied topically. Not much used but found in some analgesic mixtures and in ear drops. May cause skin rashes and bone marrow suppression. Overdose may result in nausea, coma, and convulsions. The rate of metabolism (half-life) of single doses is sometimes used as a measure of drug metabolism by the liver.

Phenbenicillin. As for PHENOXYMETHYLPENICILLIN.

Phencyclidine (m). Drug of abuse commonly known as 'Angel Dust'. Originally used as an aid to anaesthesia, but found to cause pronounced psychotic effects which are usually unpleasant.

Phenelzine. Antidepressant; inhibits monoamine oxidase thus increasing tissue concentrations of NORADRENALINE, DOPAMINE, and 5-HYDROXYTRYPTAMINE. Adverse effects include hepatitis, interactions with tyramine-containing foods, and indirect sympathomimetic amines producing hypertensive crises, and with narcotics to produce profound CNS depression. Hypertensive crisis treated with alpha-adrenoceptor blocker (e.g., PHENTALOMINE).

Phenindamine. Antihistamine, with actions and uses similar to PROMETHAZINE. Unlike most antihistamines, it causes stimulant side effects and may be used when sedation is a problem. May cause insomnia, convulsions, dry mouth, and gastro-intestinal disturbances.

Phenindione. Anticoagulant, with actions and interactions similar to WARFARIN. Adverse effects include allergic reactions, jaundice, and steatorrhoea.

Pheniramine. Antihistamine, with actions, uses, and adverse effects similar to PROMETHAZINE.

Phenmetrazine (c). Anorectic/sympathomimetic amine, widely abused, with actions and adverse effects of AMPHETAMINE.

Phenobarbital. rINN for PHENOBARBITONE.

Phenobarbitone (c). (Phenobarbital–USA). Long-acting barbiturate anticonvulsant. Depresses epileptic discharges in the brain. Used orally as preventive treatment in epileptics and occasionally by injection to control a severe fit. Danger of sedation and impairment of learning capacity. Induces its own metabolism by the liver. Given only with caution in liver disease. Danger of drug interaction. Coma with respiratory depression in overdose. No antidote. Treatment is supportive, sometimes plus forced alkaline diuresis or haemodialysis to promote excretion of the drug.

Phenol. Disinfectant in dilute solution; in strong solutions it denatures cell proteins and damages sensory nerves. Uses include injection for the sclerosis of haemorrhoids and alleviation of intractable pain by localized effects in the nerves involved.

Phenolphthalein. Purgative that acts by direct stimulation of colonic muscle. Action prolonged by absorption of drug from the gut and recirculation in bile. Produces pink urine and faeces (red if alkaline). May cause skin rashes in sensitive individuals.

Phenoperidine (c). Narcotic analgesic, with actions and adverse effects similar to MORPHINE. Used with DROPERIDOL to produce neuroleptanalgesia – a state of consciousness but calmness and indifference – allowing the patient to cooperate with the surgeon.

Phenothrin. Synthetic pyrethroid insecticide used for topical application against head-lice. Active against lice and eggs. Shampoo is irritant to eyes but systemic toxicity is unlikely.

Phenoxybenzamine. Alkylating agent with alpha-adrenoceptor blocking and antihistamine effects. Used in phaeochromocytoma. Side effects include sedation, nausea, and vomiting.

Phenoxybenzylpenicillin (Phenbenicillin). As for PHENOXYMETHYLPENICILLIN.

Phenoxyethylpenicillin (Phenethicillin). As for PHENOXYMETHYLPENICILLIN.

Phenoxymethylpenicillin (Penicillin V). Acid-resistant PENICILLIN used orally. Shares actions and adverse effects of BENZYLPENICILLIN.

Phenoxypropanol. Preservative/anti-infective for skin preparations.

Phenoxypropylpenicillin (Propicillin). As for PHENOXYMETHYLPENICILLIN.

Phensuximide. Anticonvulsant essentially similar to ETHOSUXIMIDE.

Phentermine (c). Anorectic/sympathomimetic amine. Actions and adverse effects similar to DIETHYLPROPION.

Phentolamine. Alpha-adrenoceptor blocking drug with partial agonist and smooth muscle relaxant activity. Used in phaeochromocytoma to manage high blood pressure and as a diagnostic test. May be used with PAPAVERINE in erectile impotence. Side effects include tachycardia, gastro-intestinal disturbance and nasal stuffiness.

Phenylbutazone. Anti-inflammatory/analgesic used in treatment of inflammatory joint disorders. Adverse effects include nausea, vomiting, skin rashes, peptic ulceration, sodium retention, and hypotension. Occasionally causes bone marrow depression with thrombocytopaenia, agranulocytosis, and aplastic anaemia. May enhance action of oral anticoagulants (e.g., WARFARIN). Owing to high incidence of adverse effects, its use has been restricted to one condition only, ankylosing spondylitis.

Phenylephrine. Sympathomimetic amine, with actions, uses, and toxicity of NORADRENALINE. Also used as mydriatic and nasal decongestant.

Phenylpropanolamine (m). Sympathomimetic, with actions, uses, and adverse effects similar to EPHEDRINE.

Phenytoin. Anticonvulsant. Suppresses epileptic discharge in the brain. Used orally to prevent convulsions and by injection to control convulsions or to suppress irregular heart rhythms. Long-term use may cause gum hypertrophy, acne, hirsutism, folate deficiency, anaemia, osteomalacia, and liver enzyme induction with danger of drug interactions. In mild overdosage, causes ataxia, dysarthria, and nystagmus. Coma and respiratory depression occur in severe cases. No antidote; supportive therapy only.

Pholcodine. Narcotic derivative related to CODEINE but with little analgesic activity. Used only for cough suppression. May cause constipation. Similar to CODEINE in overdosage.

Phosphoric acid. In dilute form acts as a stimulant to gastric secretion.

Phosphorylcolamine. Synthetic amino acid with high phosphorus content. Said to promote improved metabolism. Used as a 'tonic' in debilitated patients.

Physostigmine (Eserine). Anticholinesterase, allowing accumulation of ACETYLCHOLINE. Actions those of ACETYLCHOLINE. Effects of overdose antagonized by ATROPINE.

Phytomenadione. *See* VITAMIN K.

Pilocarpine. Parasympathomimetic drug, with actions of ACETYLCHOLINE. Used as eye drops in the treatment of glaucoma where it reduces ocular pressure by constricting the pupils to improve drainage. Also used to stimulate saliva production in cases of xerstomia (dry mouth) after radiotherapy.

Pimozide. Tranquillizer, with uses, adverse effects, etc. similar to CHLORPROMAZINE.

Pindolol. Beta-adrenoceptor blocking drug with partial agonist activity (intrinsic sympathomimetic activity). Uses, side effects, etc. as for PROPRANOLOL.

Pipenzolate. Anticholinergic, with actions and adverse effects similar to ATROPINE. Used to reduce gastric acid secretion and intestinal spasm.

Piperacillin. Broad-spectrum, injectable PENICILLIN similar to CARBENICILLIN, particularly effective against gram-negative organisms including *Pseudomonas*, *Proteus*, anaerobes. Used in severe, life-threatening infections. Adverse effects include pseudomembranous colitis, leucopenia and interstitial nephritis. Dosage reduction needed in renal failure.

Piperazine. Used in treatment of threadworms and roundworms. Adverse effects include dizziness and ataxia.

Pipothiazine. Phenothiazine tranquillizer, with indications, actions, and adverse effects similar to FLUPHENAZINE.

Pipotiazine. rINN for PIPOTHIAZINE.

Piracetam. Anticonvulsant used as an adjunct to other drug treatment in cortical myoclonus (spontaneous disabling jerking movements associated with an epileptic focus in the brain). May cause abnormal movements, insomnia, nervousness, drowsiness, depression and weight gain.

Pirbuterol. Bronchoselective beta-adrenoceptor agonist, with actions, uses, and adverse effects similar to SALBUTAMOL.

Pirenzepine. Anticholinergic with selective effects on gastric mucosa. Reduces gastric acid secretion while causing less of the adverse effects normally associated with such compounds (*see* ATROPINE). May cause dry mouth and blurred vision.

Piretanide. Diuretic, with actions, uses, and adverse effects similar to FRUSEMIDE.

Piroxicam. Non-steroid anti-inflammatory/analgesic with long duration of action needing only once daily dosage. Actions and uses similar to IBUPROFEN. Adverse effects include gastro-intestinal intolerance and oedema.

Pituitary gland extract. Extract of animal pituitary tissue used for its antidiuretic activity. *See* VASOPRESSIN.

Pivampicillin. Prodrug antibiotic. Readily absorbed from gastro-intestinal tract and rapidly metabolized to the active drug AMPICILLIN, whose actions, uses, and adverse effects it shares.

Pivmecillinam. Prodrug antibiotic. Readily absorbed from gastro-intestinal tract and rapidly metabolized to the active drug MECILLINAM, whose actions, uses, and adverse effects it shares.

Pizotifen. For prevention of migraine. Has antiserotonin and antihistamine properties. May cause drowsiness, weight gain, dizziness, and nausea.

Podophyllin. Plant extract resin, with antimitotic and purgative actions. Used topically to treat warts and by mouth as an irritant purgative (mainly succeeded by less irritant compounds).

Podophyllotoxin. Purified extract of PODOPHYLLUM used to treat genital warts. Local adverse effects are fewer and milder compared with PODOPHYLLIN. May cause local irritation.

Podophyllum. Purgative. Pronounced irritant effect on the bowel or skin. Because of its violent effects has been replaced by milder drugs. Still used as a paint for warts where it prevents growth.

Poldine. Parasympatholytic, with actions, etc. similar to ATROPINE. Used to reduce gastric acid secretion in treatment of peptic ulceration.

Poloxalene. Purgative. Lowers surface tension of intestinal fluids and softens faeces.

Poloxamer '188'. *See* POLOXALENE.

Polyacrylic acid. Gel used as a tear fluid substitute for management of dry eye conditions.

Polyethylene glycol. Used as a solvent and/or moisturizing agent in topical preparations.

Polymyxin B. Antibiotic active against gram-negative bacteria. Not absorbed when taken by mouth but effective topically (e.g., within gut or on skin or eyes). May also be given by intramuscular injection. Rarely causes skin sensitivity but injections may be painful and associated with neurological symptoms.

Polynoxylin. Antiseptic, with wide antibacterial and antifungal actions. Used topically for skin, throat, and external ear infections.

Polyoestradiol. Sex hormone. Used in treatment of carcinoma of the prostate. Adverse effects similar to ETHINYLOESTRADIOL.

Polysaccharide–iron complex. Haematinic, with actions, uses, and adverse effects similar to FERROUS SULPHATE.

Polysorbate 60. Emulsifying agent. Aids water-in-oil mixtures and solubilizing of fat-soluble substances.

Polythiazide. Thiazide diuretic similar to BENDROFLUAZIDE.

Polyvinyl alcohol. A synthetic resin with strong hydrophilic properties used in eye drops to lubricate dry eyes and in jelly skin preparations which dry rapidly to form a soluble plastic film.

Poractant. Extract from porcine lung used to treat lung damage (Respiratory Distress Syndrome) in preterm infants. Similar to COLFOSCERIL.

Posterior pituitary extract. Mixed hormonal extract, with actions of OXYTOCIN and VASOPRESSIN whose toxic effects it also shares. Used by injection or nasal absorption to treat diabetes insipidus.

Potassium aluminium sulphate. *See* ALUM.

Potassium benzoate. Used topically for mild fungal infections of the skin: *see* BENZOIC ACID. Also used in mixtures of potassium salts for oral treatment of potassium deficiency.

Potassium bicarbonate. Antacid. Has been used as gastric antacid as SODIUM BICARBONATE, but unsuitable for intravenous use.

Potassium canrenoate. Potassium-sparing diuretic, related to, and with similar actions, uses, and adverse effects to SPIRONOLACTONE.

Potassium chloride. Potassium supplement. Used when there is a danger of hypokalaemia (e.g., treatment with potassium-losing diuretics) and fluid overload in liver failure. Oral potassium chloride itself causes nausea and gastric irritation. Usually administered as slow-release preparation or in an effervescent solution of bicarbonate and trimethylglycine. May be given by slow intravenous infusion. Danger of hyperkalaemia in renal failure. Treated by haemodialysis and ion exchange resins.

Potassium citrate. Renders urine less acid. Used to reduce bladder inflammation. May produce adverse effects similar to POTASSIUM CHLORIDE.

Potassium glycerophosphate. A source of additional dietary potassium and phosphate used in 'tonics'.

Potassium *para*-aminobenzoate. Nutrient. *See para-*AMINOBENZOIC ACID. Has been used to treat skin disorders where there is excessive fibrosis (e.g., scleroderma).

Potassium perchlorate. Treatment for overactive thyroid gland. Reduces formation of thyroid hormone by interfering with uptake of iodine into the gland. May cause nausea, vomiting, rashes, kidney damage, and bone marrow suppression.

Povidone-iodine. Antiseptic. Liberates inorganic iodine slowly on to the skin or mucous membranes. Used pre-operatively and in treatment of wounds.

Practolol. Cardioselective beta-adrenoceptor blocking drug. Withdrawn because of adverse effects on eye, ear, and peritoneum.

Pralidoxime (P2S). Cholinesterase reactivator used in treatment of organophosphorus cholinesterase poisoning.

Pramocaine. rINN for PRAMOXINE.

Pramoxine. Surface-active local anaesthetic, with actions and adverse effects similar to LIGNOCAINE. Used topically on skin or mucous membranes.

Pravastatin. Enzyme inhibitor which reduces blood cholesterol formation when diet alone is not effective. Actions similar to SIMVASTATIN. Adverse effects include rash, myalgia, headache, chest pain, gastrointestinal disturbances and fatigue.

Praziquantel. Anti-infective for treatment of schistosomiasis. Active against *S. haematobium* and *S. japonicum.* Effective both in urinary tract and hepatic infections. Adverse effects, usually transient, include nausea, epigastric pain, dizziness, and drowsiness.

Prazosin. Vasodilator/antihypertensive. Adverse effects include tachycardia and headache. Excessive fall in blood pressure may occur early in treatment.

Prednisolone. Synthetic CORTICOSTEROID, with actions, etc. as for PREDNISONE.

Prednisone. Synthetic CORTICOSTEROID, with similar actions, etc. to CORTISONE, but has greater anti-inflammatory activity with less salt and water retention.

Prenalterol. Synthetic beta-adrenoceptor agonist which increases the force of cardiac contraction with only minor increases in heart rate and little, if any, peripheral vascular actions. Used in intractable heart failure. May be useful as antidote in overdosage of beta-adrenoceptor antagonists.

Prenylamine. Vasodilator used to prevent angina attacks. May cause gastro-intestinal symptoms, flushing, skin rashes, and hypotension. Contraindicated in cardiac or liver failure.

Prilocaine. Local anaesthetic similar to LIGNOCAINE, but less toxic. Used in dentistry.

Primaquine. Antimalarial agent. Adverse effects include nausea, methaemoglobinaemia, and haemolytic anaemia.

Primidone. Anticonvulsant. Similar to barbiturates; partly metabolized by liver to PHENOBARBITONE. Suppresses epileptic discharges in the brain. Used orally to prevent convulsions. Additive effect with PHENOBARBITONE, to which it is otherwise essentially similar.

Probenecid. For prevention of gout. Increases urine excretion of uric acid and thus reduces its levels in the body. May cause nausea, vomiting, and skin rashes. Reduces excretion of PENICILLIN.

Probucol. Reduces elevated concentrations of serum cholesterol with lesser effect on triglycerides. Used in hypercholesterolaemia.

Procainamide. Antidysrhythmic/local anaesthetic similar to PROCAINE but longer-acting and with less CNS stimulation. Used to treat cardiac dysrhythmias, but contraindicated in heart block. May cause dose-related hypotension, mental depression, and hallucinations. Hypersensitivity may cause arthritis and rash (systemic lupus erythematosus-like syndrome).

Procaine. Local anaesthetic. Stabilizes nerve cell membranes to prevent impulse transmission. Used by injection for anaesthesia in minor operations. Poor activity if applied topically. Short action (due to rapid removal in the blood) may be prolonged by combination with a vasoconstrictor (e.g., ADRENALINE). May cause CNS stimulation with euphoria and convulsions. Metabolite of procaine interferes with antimicrobial activity of sulphonamides (e.g., SULPHADIMIDINE). Preparations containing adrenaline are contraindicated in heart disease, hyperthyroidism, or treatment with tricyclic antidepressants (e.g., AMITRIPTYLINE) where it may cause cardiac dysrhythmias.

Procaine benylpenicillin. rINN for PROCAINE PENICILLIN.

Procaine penicillin. Long-acting form of BENZYLPENICILLIN, with similar actions and adverse effects.

Procarbazine. Cytotoxic drug used in neoplastic disease. Adverse effects include nausea, vomiting, diarrhoea, stomatitis, alopecia, neurotoxicity, and bone marrow depression.

Prochlorperazine. Phenothiazine similar to CHLORPROMAZINE, but less sedative and more potent antiemetic actions. Used mainly as an antiemetic. More likely than CHLORPROMAZINE to cause extrapyramidal side effects. May be given orally, by buccal absorption, by injection, or as a suppository.

Procyclidine. Parasympatholytic used in treatment of parkinsonism. Actions, etc. similar to BENZHEXOL.

Progesterone. Sex hormone acts on the uterus (in sequence with OESTROGEN) to prepare the endometrium to receive the fertilized ovum. Has been used in treatment of uterine bleeding, for contraception, for breast and uterine tumours, and for threatened abortion. In low doses used as a hormone supplement to treat menstrual disorders, premenstrual syndrome and infertility. Has to be injected and therefore largely replaced by newer progestational agents which are active by mouth. May cause acne, weight gain, enlargement of the breasts, headache, gastro-intestinal symptoms, ovarian cysts and jaundice.

Proguanil. Antimalarial agent. Adverse effects include vomiting and renal irritation.

Prolintane. CNS stimulant claimed to have effect intermediate between CAFFEINE and AMPHETAMINE. Used to treat lethargy. May cause nausea, rapid heart rate, and insomnia.

Promazine. Phenothiazine/antihistamine similar to CHLORPROMAZINE.

Promethazine. Phenothiazine/antihistamine with actions similar to CHLORPROMAZINE. Used as an antiemetic and in treatment of allergic reactions, but has little antipsychotic effects. Marked sedative effects make it useful as a hypnotic in children and in pre-operative medication. Adverse effects and overdosage effects similar to CHLORPROMAZINE.

Propafenone. Antiarrhythmic used to prevent and treat life-threatening irregular cardiac rhythms.

Propamidine. Antiseptic, with antibacterial and antifungal actions. Used topically for infections of skin and conjunctiva. Treatment should not be prolonged more than one week or tissue damage may occur.

Propantheline. Parasympatholytic, with peripheral and toxic effects similar to ATROPINE. Used to reduce gastric acid secretion in peptic ulceration and as an antispasmodic for gastro-intestinal and urinary complaints. Contraindications and overdosage effects as for ATROPINE.

Propicillin. Essentially similar to PHENOXYMETHYLPENICILLIN.

Propranolol. Beta-adrenoceptor antagonist used in angina, hypertension, arrhythmias, hyperthyroidism, migraine, anxiety and to prevent recurrence of myocardial infarction. May cause bronchoconstriction, cardiac failure, cold extremities, and sleep disturbances.

Propylene glycol. Solvent used in extract of some crude drugs and as a vehicle for some injections and topical applications. May cause local irritation but less toxic than other glycols owing to rapid breakdown and excretion.

Propylhexedrine. Sympathomimetic used as inhalation for treatment of nasal congestion. Actions and adverse effects similar to NAPHAZOLINE.

Propylthiouracil. Depresses formation of thyroid hormone. Used in treatment of hyperthyroidism. Adverse effects include allergic rashes, headache, nausea, diarrhoea, and blood dyscrasias, including tendency to bleeding.

Prostacyclin. *See* EPOPROSTENOL.

Protamine sulphate. Specific antidote to anticoagulant effect of HEPARIN. Derived from fish protein. Adverse effects include hypotension and dyspnoea.

Prothionamide. Anti-tuberculous agent, with actions and uses similar to ETHIONAMIDE. May be better tolerated.

Protionamide. rINN for PROTHIONAMIDE.

Protirelin. Also known as thyrotrophin-releasing-hormone (TRH). Used intravenously as a diagnostic agent in difficult cases of hypothyroidism where it causes a rapid rise of plasma THYROTROPHIN (TSH) in normal cases.

Protriptyline. Antidepressant, with similar action and adverse effects to IMIPRAMINE but has central stimulating effects. Used to treat depression associated with withdrawal and lack of energy. May aggravate anxiety and insomnia.

Proxymetacaine. Surface-active, local anaesthetic with actions and adverse effects similar to LIGNOCAINE. Used in ophthalmology.

Pseudoephedrine (m). Sympathomimetic, with actions, uses, and adverse effects similar to EPHEDRINE. Used mainly as decongestant. Said to have less effect on increasing blood pressure.

Psilocybin (m). The hallucinogenic alkaloid obtained from *Psilocybe semilanceate,* the Liberty cap mushroom or 'magic mushroom', and from related species. Metabolized to the active compound psilocin. Actions and adverse effects similar to LSD but of shorter duration.

Psyllium. Purgative. Increases faecal bulk by same mechanism as METHYLCELLULOSE.

Pumactant. Synthetic, protein-free, pulmonary surfactant administered into the airways to treat the surfactant deficiency which is the cause of Respiratory Distress Syndrome in premature babies. Surfactant (natural or synthetic) coats the airways and reduces surface tension at the air/alveoli interface thus making easier the mechanical effort involved in breathing. Used as an adjunct to artificial ventilation.

Pyrantel. Antiworm treatment. Acts by paralysing mature and immature forms, thus allowing their excretion. Little absorbed from the gut so that its activity is concentrated where needed at the site of the infection. Used as a single dose for threadworm, hookworm, roundworm, whipworm and trichostrongyliasis. May cause gastro-intestinal disturbances, headache, dizziness, drowsiness, insomnia, and rashes.

Pyrazinamide. Anti-tuberculous drug. High incidence of adverse effects, particularly liver toxicity.

Pyridostigmine. Anticholinesterase, with actions similar to PHYSOSTIGMINE.

Pyridoxine (Vitamin B_6). Vitamin used in treatment of specific deficiency and other anaemias and in ISONIAZID-induced neuropathy. Recommended also for depression due to the oral contraceptive but true pyridoxine deficiency is not universal in such cases.

Pyrimethamine. Antimalarial agent. Adverse effects include skin rashes and folate-deficient anaemia.

Q

Quetiapine. Antipsychotic/tranquillizer with actions and uses similar to CLOZAPINE. Does not appear to cause bone marrow depression but may cause drowsiness, dry mouth, dizziness and constipation.

Quinagolide. Dopamine antagonist. Suppresses hyper-prolactinaemia and thus can be used to stop galactorrhoea and to assist return to a normal menstrual cycle and normal fertility. Adverse effects include nausea, vomiting, other gastro-intestinal effects, headache, and hypotension.

Quinalbarbitone (c). Barbiturate hypnotic usually prescribed in combined preparation with AMYLOBARBITONE. No major differences from AMYLOBARBITONE.

Quinapril. Antihypertensive with actions, uses and adverse effects similar to CAPTOPRIL.

Quinidine. Antidysrhythmic agent, with local anaesthetic activity. Depresses myocardial contractility and impulse conduction. Reduces cardiac output. Used to prevent recurrent dysrhythmias or to convert established dysrhythmias back to normal sinus rhythm. Dose-dependent effects include vertigo, tinnitus, deafness, blurred vision, confusion, gastro-intestinal symptoms, cardiac arrhythmias, and cardiac arrest. Rashes and bruising are dose-independent. Contraindicated when dysrhythmia is due to DIGOXIN or when there is heart block.

Quinine. Antimalarial agent. Used to reduce skeletal muscle spasms. Adverse effects include vomiting, psychosis, visual and auditory disturbances, haemolytic anaemia, and thrombocytopenia. Toxic doses may cause abortion.

R

Raltitrexed. Cytotoxic used in palliative treatment of large bowel (colorectal) cancer. May cause gastro-intestinal disorders, bone marrow suppression, CNS symptoms, muscle pains, weakness and hair loss.

Ramipril. Antihypertensive with actions, uses and adverse effects similar to CAPTOPRIL. A pro-drug which is converted to Ramiprilat before exerting its effect.

Ranitidine. Selectively blocks histamine receptors mediating gastric acid secretions. Uses and adverse effects similar to CIMETIDINE, but may cause less CNS effects or breast enlargement in males. Has fewer interactions with other drugs.

Ranitidine bismuth citrate. A complex of ranitidine and bismuth for treatment of peptic ulcers. May be used in combination with antibiotics in patients with *Helicobacter pylori* infection. Ranitidine reduces gastric acid secretions by selectively blocking histamine receptors and bismuth inhibits growth of *H. pylori* and has antacid properties. May cause blackening of tongue and stools, gastro-intestinal disturbance and headache. Prolonged use may allow sufficient absorption of bismuth to cause kidney damage, liver damage and CNS effects.

Rauwolfia. Indian shrub. *See* RESERPINE for main derivative.

Razoxane. Antimitotic used in treatment of certain bone and soft-tissue tumours together with radiotherapy. May cause gastro-intestinal disturbance, bone marrow suppression, and hair loss.

Reboxetine. Selective NORADRENALINE reuptake blocker used in the treatment of depression. Less likely to cause troublesome anticholinergic effects than the TRICYCLIC ANTIDEPRESSANTS but may cause dry mouth, constipation, insomnia, sweating, palpitations, urinary retention and impotence.

Remifentanil. Short acting opioid analgesic similar to FENTANYL and ALFENTANIL. Used in induction and maintenance of anaesthesia. The short action allows for more rapid recovery after surgery. May cause respiratory depression, bradycardia, nausea and vomiting.

Remoxipride. Antipsychotic, with actions and uses similar to CHLORPROMAZINE. Adverse effects include sedation, involuntary movements, agitation, and anticholinergic effects. Withdrawn due to risk of bone marrow suppression (aplastic anaemia).

Reproterol. Beta-adrenoceptor agonist, with actions, uses, and adverse effects as for SALBUTAMOL.

Reserpine. Rauwolfia derivative. Reduces sympathetic tone by NORADRENALINE depletion. Depletes brain NORADRENALINE, DOPAMINE, and 5-HYDROXYTRYPTAMINE. Used in hypertension and as antipsychotic. Adverse effects include depression, parkinsonism, nasal stuffiness, fluid retention, and impotence.

Resorcinol. Dermatological treatment. Reduces itching and helps remove scaly skin. Used topically in treatment of acne and dandruff. Also as ear drops where used for antiseptic effects. If absorbed over long term, may cause suppression of thyroid gland. If ingested, is corrosive and may cause kidney damage, coma, and convulsions.

Retinol. *See* VITAMIN A.

Ribavirin. Antiviral agent. Administered by inhalation to treat infants and children with severe chest infection caused by the respiratory syncytial virus (RSV).

Riboflavin. rINN for RIBOFLAVINE.

Riboflavine (Vitamin B_2). Vitamin. Deficiency leads to mucosal ulceration and angular stomatitis.

Ricinoleic acid. Acid that forms stable soaps with alkalis. Used in contraceptive creams and jellies.

Rifabutin. Antibiotic used prophylactically to prevent infection with tuberculosis and related organisms in patients with impaired immunity. Adverse effects include anaemia, gastro-intestinal disturbances and discolouration of skin, urine and body secretions.

Rifampicin. Bactericidal antibiotic, used in tuberculosis. Adverse effects include liver toxicity and influenza-like symptoms. Induces liver enzymes, so reducing effectiveness of some other drugs including oral contraceptives and corticosteroids.

Riluzole. Reduces glutamate levels in the CNS and thus protects vulnerable neurones in Motor Neurone Disease where it is used prophylactically. May cause gastro-intestinal disturbance, headache and dizziness.

Rimiterol. Beta-adrenoceptor agonist. Actions, uses, and adverse effects as for SALBUTAMOL.

Risperidone. Antipsychotic used in schizophrenia. Effective against both positive and negative symptoms e.g., delusions and poverty of speech respectively. Acts as antagonist against dopaminergic, adrenergic and 5HT receptors. Said to be well tolerated but may cause postural hypotension, extrapyramidal disturbances and other adverse effects associated with antipsychotic drugs e.g., CHLORPROMAZINE.

Ritodrine. Beta-adrenoceptor agonist. Actions, uses, and adverse effects as for ISOXSUPRINE.

Rivastigmine. Anticholinesterase inhibitor used to increase brain cholinergic activity in patients with Alzheimer's dementia. Low peripheral anticholinesterase activity improves tolerance but may still cause gastrointestinal disturbance, anorexia, weight loss, tremor, confusion and depression.

Rocuronium. Non-depolarizing skeletal muscle relaxant used as an adjunct to anaesthesia. Actions, uses and adverse effects similar to TUBOCURARINE.

Ropinirole. Dopamine agonist used to treat the dopamine deficiency in Parkinson's disease, where its effects are similar to BROMOCRIPTINE. May cause nausea, vomiting, drowsiness, hypotension and bradycardia.

Ropivacaine. Local anaesthetic similar to LIGNOCAINE and BUPIVACAINE but with more prolonged effects.

Rose bengal. Staining agent. Used for detection of damage to the cornea.

Rubella vaccine. Live attenuated rubella virus for immunization against rubella (German measles). Used routinely in girls before puberty. May be used in non-pregnant women of childbearing age. Adverse effects include rash, fever, enlarged lymph glands, joint pains. Must not be given to pregnant women or those receiving drugs to suppress the immune response.

Rubidomycin. *See* DAUNORUBICIN.

S

Salbutamol. Bronchoselective beta-adrenoceptor agonist used in bronchial asthma by inhalation, intravenous infusion or orally. Used also by intravenous infusion or orally to inhibit premature labour. Adverse effects include tachycardia, arrhythmias, tremors, and muscle cramps.

Salcatonin. Synthetic CALCITONIN hormone which regulates plasma calcium concentrations. Used short term to lower high calcium levels in Paget's disease of bone and metastatic cancer. Also used for pain relief. Adverse effects include gastro-intestinal disturbances, skin rashes, dizziness. Anaphylactic reactions have been reported.

Salicylamide. Analgesic/antipyretic, with actions and adverse effects similar to ACETYLSALICYLIC ACID but less effective and used only infrequently. In overdosage, does not cause acidosis but depression of respiration and loss of consciousness.

Salicylic acid. Anti-inflammatory/analgesic; an active metabolite of ACETYLSALICYLIC ACID whose adverse effects it shares. Not used systemically as it causes marked gastric irritation. Topically on skin it acts as a keratolytic and has bacteriostatic and anti-fungal properties. Used to treat warts, skin ulcers, psoriasis, and other skin conditions.

Salmeterol. A bronchoselective beta-adrenoceptor agonist used in bronchial asthma and chronic obstructive pulmonary disease, similar to SALBUTAMOL but with a longer duration of action. May also inhibit the underlying inflammatory disease. Adverse effects similar to SALBUTAMOL.

Salsalate. Anti-inflammatory/analgesic. After absorption is broken down to SALICYLIC ACID. Uses and adverse effects similar to ACETYLSALICYLIC ACID.

Saquinavir. Antiviral agent active against HIV. Used in combination with other antivirals in progressive disease (AIDS). May cause rash, headaches, gastro-intestinal disturbance and peripheral nerve damage.

Secobarbital. rINN for QUINALBARBITONE

Selegiline. Selective monoamine oxidase inhibitor, which prevents breakdown of DOPAMINE in the brain and so increases and prolongs the action of LEVODOPA. Used in conjunction with LEVODOPA in the treatment of Parkinson's disease. Adverse effects include hypotension, nausea, vomiting, confusion, agitation, and involuntary movements.

Selenium sulphide. Reduces formation of dandruff and other forms of eczema of the scalp. Used as a shampoo. Highly toxic if ingested causing anorexia, garlic breath, vomiting, anaemia, and liver damage.

Senna (m). Plant extract purgative, with actions, adverse effects, etc. as for CASCARA.

Sennosides A and B. Active principles of SENNA.

Sermorelin. Synthetic growth hormone releasing factor. Used intravenously as a diagnostic agent in investigation of function of the anterior pituitary gland.

Serotonin. *See* 5-HYDROXYTRYPTAMINE.

Sertindole. Antipsychotic with actions similar to CLOZAPINE but thought to be free of its adverse effects on the bone marrow. Used to treat schizophrenia. May cause nasal congestion, dizziness, weight gain, fluid retention and shortness of breath.

Sertraline. Antidepressant similar to FLUVOXAMINE which acts by blocking reuptake of serotonin into nerve cells. Unlike tricyclic antidepressants it does not cause anticholinergic or cardiac side effects. The most common side effects are dry mouth, gastro-intestinal disturbances, tremor and male sexual dysfunction.

Silver nitrate. Disinfectant/cleansing agent, used in wet dressings or baths for suppurating lesions. Must only be used short-term. The lotion should not be used if a precipitate is present.

Silver protein. Has mild antibacterial properties. Used in eye drops or nasal sprays for treatment of minor infections.

Silver sulphadiazine. Sulphonamide derivative, with actions similar to SULPHADIMIDINE. Used topically in treatment of burns to prevent infection.

Simvastatin. Reduces blood levels of cholesterol when diet alone is not effective. Inhibits the synthesis of cholesterol without reducing uptake into cells. Adverse effects include gastro-intestinal disturbance, tiredness, rashes, myalgia and muscle weakness.

Soap spirit. Soft soap in alcohol used in some dermatological preparations for its cleaning and descaling actions.

Sodium acid citrate. Anticoagulant. Now preferred to SODIUM CITRATE.

Sodium acid phosphate. Saline purgative, with actions and uses similar to SODIUM PHOSPHATE.

Sodium alkyl sulphoacetate. Wetting agent/laxative. Used mainly as an enema for treatment of persistent constipation and pre-operative bowel evacuation.

Sodium antimonylgluconate (Triostam). Used in schistosomiasis. Adverse effects include anorexia, nausea, vomiting, diarrhoea, muscle and joint pains, and cardiotoxicity.

Sodium aurothiomalate. Gold salt, used in rheumatic diseases, notably severe rheumatoid arthritis where it is capable of halting the disease process. Given intramuscularly in weekly doses, it takes up to four to six months to achieve maximum effect. Adverse effects include mouth ulcers, skin rashes, oedema, proteinuria, blood dyscrasias, colitis, peripheral neuritis, and pulmonary fibrosis. The high incidence of adverse effects can be reduced if use of this drug is controlled from specialist rheumatology centres.

Sodium bicarbonate. Absorbable (systemic) antacid. Rapidly dissolves and neutralizes acid in stomach. Produces quick relief of dyspepsia due to peptic ulceration but is not retained in stomach and therefore has short duration of action. Absorbed from small intestine, may cause systemic alkalosis. If used in large doses, with large doses of milk may cause renal damage (i.e. 'milk–alkali syndrome'). Danger of fluid retention in patients with cardiac failure or renal disease.

Sodium calcium edetate. Chelating agent. Exchanges its calcium for other metal ions in the blood. Most effective exchange is for lead and it may be used by injection or by mouth for treatment of lead poisoning. May cause nausea, diarrhoea, abdominal cramps, and pain and thrombophlebitis at site of injection. Renal damage and dermatitis have occurred with prolonged treatment. Used with caution if there is pre-existing renal disease.

Sodium cellulose phosphate. Non-absorbable powder taken by mouth in treatment of hypercalcaemia. Adsorbs calcium ions in the intestine and prevents their absorption thus reducing the dietary intake of calcium.

Sodium chloride. Essential component of body fluids and tissues. Used intravenously to replace lost fluids when rapid treatment is needed or orally when replacement is less urgent (e.g., for sweat loss in tropics). Hyperosmolar solutions have been recommended as an emetic for first-aid treatment of poisoning, but saline is a poor emetic and may cause death due to hypernatraemia. This use is no longer recommended.

Sodium citrate. Mild purgative used in some enemas. Was used as an anticoagulant in blood for transfusion but now superseded by SODIUM ACID CITRATE. Used as alkalizing agent in treatment of cystitis.

Sodium clodronate. Acts on bone mineral metabolism to suppress bone reabsorption without affecting absorption. Used in malignant disease to treat hypercalcaemia caused by bone dissolution. Adverse effects include gastro-intestinal upsets and occasionally hypocalcaemia.

Sodium cromoglicate. rINN for SODIUM CROMOGLYCATE.

Sodium cromoglycate. Preventive treatment for asthma, rhinitis (hay fever), and conjunctivitis due to allergy. Also used for ulcerative colitis. Acts by blocking allergic mechanisms. Administered orally, by inhalation of powder or topically in eye. May cause bronchial irritation and spasm, and contact dermatitis.

Sodium edetate. Chelating agent used intravenously to reduce high blood calcium levels. Actions and adverse effects similar to SODIUM CALCIUM EDETATE. May cause excessive lowering of calcium levels.

Sodium fluoride. Used for the prevention of dental caries in areas where the intake of fluoride from drinking water is low. May be given in water or fruit juice or applied to the teeth in solution or toothpaste. Adverse effects occur only in overdosage or from high environmental fluoride levels. Large overdoses may cause gastro-intestinal symptoms, paralysis and convulsions, with death from cardiac and respiratory failure. Chronic poisoning may cause increased bone density and eye damage.

Sodium glycerophosphate. A source of additional dietary sodium and phosphate used in 'tonics'.

Sodium hyaluronate. Transparent, high-viscosity sodium salt of high-molecular-weight carbohydrate. Used in ophthalmic surgery to replace aqueous and vitreous humour.

Sodium hypochlorite. Source of chlorine, which has antimicrobial action for cleansing and desloughing of skin ulcers.

Sodium iodide. Expectorant. Causes increased and more watery bronchial secretion. Included in some cough mixtures. Acts also as a source of iodine (essential for production of thyroid hormone). Added to table salt to prevent endemic goitre and may be used preoperatively to prepare hyperactive goitre for removal. Should not be given in pulmonary tuberculosis where it may reactivate the disease.

Sodium iron edetate. Haematinic, with actions, uses, and adverse effects similar to FERROUS SULPHATE.

Sodium lactate. Salt administered intravenously to increase the alkali reserve. Metabolized to bicarbonate. Contraindicated in liver failure, where conversion to bicarbonate is impaired.

Sodium lauryl sulphate. Detergent/wetting agent. Used for cleaning properties in skin preparations and in enemas to aid softening of faeces.

Sodium lauryl sulphoacetate. Similar to SODIUM LAURYL SULPHATE.

Sodium morrhuate. Sclerosing agent used for injection treatment of varicose veins; causes obliteration of the dilated vessels. May cause allergic reactions. A test dose is recommended.

Sodium nitrite. Used in treatment of cyanide poisoning in conjunction with SODIUM THIOSULPHATE. The nitrite produces methaemoglobin which reacts with cyanide ions to produce cyanmethaemoglobin. Cyanmethaemoglobin does not damage cell respiration but slowly breaks down, releasing cyanide in smaller amounts which are converted to the less toxic thiocyanate by the thiosulphate.

Sodium nitroprusside. Potent, rapid-acting antihypertensive used by intravenous infusion for severe hypertensive crisis or for controlled hypotension during surgical procedures. Acts by direct dilatation of blood vessels. Duration brief as metabolized to cyanide and then thiocyanate. Adverse effects include sweating, nausea, vomiting, weakness, and muscle twitching. Excessive dosage may lead to 'cyanide poisoning' (i.e. tachycardia, hyperventilation, cardiac arrhythmias plus the above symptoms). DICOBALT EDETATE or SODIUM NITRITE plus SODIUM THIOSULPHATE are antidotes.

Sodium perborate. Mild disinfectant/deodorant used for mouth infections. Prolonged use may cause blistering and swelling in mouth.

Sodium phosphate. Saline purgative. Poorly absorbed from the gastro-intestinal tract. Retains water in the intestine and thus increases faecal mass.

Sodium picosulfate. rINN for SODIUM PICOSULPHATE.

Sodium picosulphate. Saline purgative with actions and uses similar to MAGNESIUM SULPHATE.

Sodium polystyrene sulphonate. Ion exchange resin used in treatment of high plasma potassium levels where it exchanges sodium ions for potassium. May be used orally or rectally. Adverse effects include nausea, vomiting, constipation, and sodium overload which may cause cardiac failure.

Sodium pyrrolidone-carboxylate. Hygroscopic salt. Used as a moisturing agent for dry skin.

Sodium ricinoleate. Surface-active agent used in some toothpastes for its cleaning properties.

Sodium salicylate. Analgesic/anti-inflammatory/antipyretic, with actions, uses, and adverse effects similar to ACETYLSALICYLIC ACID. Usually taken in solution. Danger of sodium overload in patients with cardiac failure or renal failure.

Sodium sulphate (Glauber's salts). Saline purgative. Actions and uses similar to MAGNESIUM SULPHATE. Unpleasant taste. Danger of sodium retention with congestive heart failure in susceptible subjects.

Sodium tetradecyl sulphate. Injection used for treatment of varicose veins.

Sodium thiosulphate. Used in treatment of cyanide poisoning together with SODIUM NITRITE.

Sodium valproate. Anticonvulsant. May act by increasing brain levels of gamma-aminobutyric acid (GABA). Used in all forms of epilepsy. May cause gastro-intestinal symptoms, liver necrosis, and prolonged bleeding times with thrombocytopenia. Before surgery, check for bleeding tendencies. May potentiate effects of antidepressant drugs whose dose should be reduced in combined treatment.

Soft paraffin. Topical emollient and protective used on skin in 'barrier creams' and wound dressings where it aids removal of the dressing.

Somatotrophin (Growth hormone). Human growth hormone. Extracted from pituitary glands. Was used to treat short stature when the epiphyses remain open.

Now withdrawn because of association with transmission of viral infections.

Somatropin. Synthetic human growth hormone produced by bacteria using recombinant DNA technology. Identical in structure to endogenous human growth hormone.

Sorbic acid. Preservative with antibacterial and antifungal properties.

Sorbide nitrate. *See* ISOSORBIDE DINITRATE.

Sorbitol. Carbohydrate poorly absorbed by mouth, but used as intravenous infusion it is a useful source of calories. May also be used as sweetening agent in diabetic foods, in dialysis fluids, and as a laxative.

Sotalol. Beta-adrenoceptor blocking drug. Uses, side effects, etc. as for PROPRANOLOL.

Soya oil. Vegetable oil used intravenously for nutrition in debilitating conditions and topically as an emollient for dry skin. Adverse effects from intravenous use include rash, fever, chills, bone marrow depression, and jaundice.

Spectinomycin. Antimicrobial active against a wide range of bacteria. Offers no advantages over other antimicrobials, except in treatment of gonorrhoea where a single injection may be adequate.

Spermicides. A number of different substances used in spermicidal contraceptives and administered topically into the vagina as jelly, cream, foaming tablet, pessary, aerosol, or film. Appear to act by reducing surface tension in the sperm cell surface and allowing osmotic imbalance to destroy the cell. Relatively ineffective contraceptives, they should be used in conjunction with a barrier contraceptive (e.g., the cap), unless the couple concerned accept the risk of pregnancy.

Spiramycin. Antibiotic with similar actions and adverse effects to ERYTHROMYCIN.

Spironolactone. Potassium-sparing diuretic. Acts by antagonism of the sodium-retaining hormone ALDOSTERONE and thus prevents exchange of sodium for potassium in the kidney tubule. Diuretic action is weak. Used when ALDOSTERONE is an important cause of fluid overload (e.g., liver cirrhosis and nephrotic syndrome). Toxic effects include headache, nausea, vomiting, and swelling of the breasts (especially in men). Danger of excessive potassium retention which, if severe, is treated with haemodialysis and ion exchange resins. Indications now limited to treatment of oedema in liver cirrhosis, nephrotic syndrome and heart failure, and primary hyperaldosteronism.

Squalane. Ingredient of skin ointments that increases skin permeability to drugs.

Squill. Expectorant. Has irritant action on gastric mucosa and produces reflex expectorant action. Used in cough mixtures for chronic bronchitis when sputum is scanty, but too irritant for use in acute bronchitis. May cause nausea, vomiting, diarrhoea, and slowing of heart rate.

Stanozolol. Sex hormone, with actions, uses, and adverse effects similar to TESTOSTERONE. Used in Behcet's disease and for prevention of hereditary angio-oedema. Long-term use may cause jaundice; used with caution in liver disease.

Starch. Polysaccharide prepared from maize, wheat, or potato. Used as an absorbent in dusting powders for skin lesions. Also used as a disintegrating agent in tablets, as a mucilage in infant feeds, and as an antidote in iodine poisoning.

Stavudine. Antiviral agent with actions against HIV. Similar to ZIDOVUDINE. Used in patients with AIDS for whom ZIDOVUDINE is inappropriate. May cause headache, malaise, skin irritation, damage to peripheral nerves and neoplasia.

Stearyl alcohol. Used in ointments and creams where its solubility aids the incorporation of water or aqueous solution.

Sterculia. Plant extract. Takes up moisture and increases faecal mass which promotes peristalsis. Used as a purgative and a bulking agent in treatment of obesity.

Stibogluconate sodium. Antimony derivative. Used in treatment of leishmaniasis. Adverse effects include nausea, vomiting, diarrhoea, muscle and joint pains, and cardiotoxicity.

Stibophen. Used in schistosomiasis. Actions and adverse effects as for SODIUM ANTIMONYLGLUCONATE.

Stilboestrol. Sex hormone, with actions, uses, and adverse effects similar to OESTRADIOL.

Storax. Balsam obtained from trunk of *Liquidambar orientalis.* Has mild antiseptic action. Used topically to assist healing of skin (e.g., for bed sores and nappy rash).

Streptodornase. Enzyme derived from streptococcal bacteria. Breaks down proteins in exudates. Used together with STREPTOKINASE to help remove clotted blood or fibrinous/purulent accumulations. Administered topically, intramuscularly or by instillation into body cavities (e.g., for haemothorax). May cause pain, fever, nausea, skin rashes, and more severe allergic reactions. If haemorrhage occurs, the treatment is as for STREPTOKINASE.

Streptokinase. Plasminogen activator/fibrinolytic agent derived from *Streptococcus.* Given intravenously in thrombotic or embolic disease. May produce allergic reactions or haemorrhage which can be reversed by an antifibrinolysin such as TRANEXAMIC ACID.

Streptomycin. Bactericidal aminoglycoside antibiotic, active against tubercle bacillus, many gram-negative and some gram-positive organisms. Poorly absorbed orally. Administered intramuscularly. Excreted mainly by kidneys, so accumulates if renal function impaired. Adverse effects include hypersensitivity reactions (particularly contact dermatitis), ototoxicity, and potentiation of neuromuscular blockade.

Styramate. Centrally acting muscle relaxant. May cause drowsiness, dizziness, and rashes.

Succinic acid. Said to promote absorption of iron from the intestine.

Succinylsulphathiazole. Sulphonamide antibacterial, with actions, etc. of SULPHADIMIDINE. Poorly absorbed. Used mainly for gut infections and sterilization of bowel prior to surgery.

Sucralfate. Aluminium–sucrose complex used for treatment of peptic ulcers. Protects gastro-duodenal mucosa by forming complex with pepsin which adheres to active ulcers. May cause constipation after prolonged use, possibly due to release of aluminium.

Sulconazole. Antifungal, with broad spectrum of activity. Used topically for fungal infections of skin (e.g., tinea, pityriasis, and candidiasis). May cause hypersensitivity reactions with itching, burning, redness, and swelling.

Sulfacetamide. rINN for SULPHACETAMIDE.

Sulfadiazine. rINN for SULPHADIAZINE.

Sulfadimidine. rINN for SULPHADIMIDINE.

Sulfadoxine. Long-acting sulphonamide antibacterial with actions, uses and adverse effects similar to SULPHADIMIDINE. Has been used in treatment of leprosy and in prevention of malaria. Mainly replaced by safer, more effective products.

Sulfaguanidine. rINN for SULPHAGUANIDINE.

Sulfamethoxazole. rINN for SULPHAMETHOXAZOLE.

Sulfametopyrazine. Sulphonamide antibacterial with actions, etc. similar to SULPHADIMIDINE. Long-acting. Side effects may be more serious than SULPHADIMIDINE.

Sulfasalazine. rINN for SULPHASALAZINE.

Sulfathiazole. rINN for SULPHATHIAZOLE.

Sulfinpyrazone. rINN for SULPHINPYRAZONE.

Sulindac. Non-steroid anti-inflammatory agent with actions, uses and adverse effects similar to IBUPROFEN.

Sulphabenzamide. Sulphonamide antibacterial with actions, uses and adverse effects similar to SULPHADIMIDINE. Now used only for topical infections (e.g., in eye or ear drops).

Sulphacarbamide. Sulphonamide antibacterial, with actions and adverse effects similar to SULPHADIMIDINE. Rapidly excreted in urine and therefore used for urinary tract infections. Crystalluria said not to occur.

Sulphacetamide. Sulphonamide antibacterial, with actions similar to SULPHADIMIDINE, but used only as eye drops for eye infections.

Sulphadiazine. Sulphonamide antibacterial, with actions, etc. similar to SULPHADIMIDINE.

Sulphadimidine. Sulphonamide antibacterial, which inhibits conversion of *para*-AMINOBENZOIC ACID to FOLIC ACID. Broad spectrum of activity. Mainly used in urinary tract infections. Adverse effects include crystalluria, skin rashes, polyarteritis, and Stevens–Johnson syndrome. May produce kernicterus in newborn. Potentiates WARFARIN by competitive displacement from plasma proteins.

Sulphaguanidine. Sulphonamide antibacterial, with actions, etc. of SULPHADIMIDINE. Poorly absorbed. Used mainly for gut infections and sterilization of bowel prior to surgery.

Sulphamethizole. Sulphonamide antibacterial, with actions, etc. similar to SULPHADIMIDINE.

Sulphamethoxazole. Sulphonamide antibacterial, with actions, etc. of SULPHADIMIDINE, but somewhat longer action.

Sulphamethoxydiazine. Sulphonamide antibacterial, with actions, etc. of SULPHADIMIDINE, but only once daily administration required.

Sulphanilamide. Sulphonamide antibacterial, with actions and adverse effects similar to SULPHADIMIDINE but more toxic.

Sulphapyridine. Sulphonamide antibacterial, with actions and adverse effects similar to SULPHADIMIDINE. Toxic effects are common and its use is generally limited to treatment of dermatitis herpetiformis and other skin conditions.

Sulphasalazine. Compound of SULPHAPYRIDINE and SALICYLIC ACID. Used in ulcerative colitis. Broken down in the intestine to SULPHAPYRIDINE and MESALAZINE, the latter being active in reducing local prostaglandin synthesis. Adverse effects as for SULPHADIMIDINE.

Sulphasomizole. Sulphonamide antibacterial, with actions, etc. of SULPHADIMIDINE, but somewhat longer action.

Sulphathiazole. Sulphonamide antibacterial, with actions, etc. of SULPHADIMIDINE.

Sulphinpyrazone. Prophylactic treatment for gout. Promotes renal excretion of urates by reducing reabsorption in renal tubules. Reduces blood uric acid levels and gradually depletes urate deposits in tissues. No value in treatment of acute gout. Reduces platelet stickiness and is used to prevent thrombosis in the coronary and cerebral circulations. May cause nausea, vomiting, and abdominal pain. May aggravate peptic ulcer and may precipitate acute gout. Long-term use may suppress bone marrow activity. Caution in renal disease and peptic ulcer. May interact to enhance actions of oral anticoagulants and oral hypoglycaemics.

Sulphormethoxine. Sulphonamide antibacterial, with actions, etc. of SULPHADIMIDINE, but only once weekly administration required.

Sulphur. Used topically in skin lotions or ointments as an antiseptic.

Sulpiride. Antipsychotic, with actions (including anti-emetic) and uses similar to CHLORPROMAZINE. Adverse effects include sedation, extrapyramidal symptoms, sleep disturbance, agitation, and hypertension.

Sulthiame. Anticonvulsant. Carbonic anhydrase inhibitor similar to ACETAZOLAMIDE. Used in prevention of epilepsy, usually in addition to other drugs. May cause paraesthesia of face and extremities, hyperventilation, and gastric upsets. Inhibits PHENYTOIN metabolism and may cause phenytoin toxicity. In overdosage causes vomiting, headache, hyperventilation, and vertigo but not coma. May cause crystalluria with renal damage which is treated by alkaline diuresis.

Sumatriptan. 5-hydroxytryptamine agonist administered orally or by subcutaneous auto-injection to relieve migraine attacks. Acts at receptors in the cranial blood vessels to reduce vasodilation associated with throbbing headache. May cause pain at the injection site, flushing, feelings of chest tightness and tiredness, and transient hypertension. Contra-indicated if there is a history of heart disease or other vascular disease.

Suramin. Anti-worm treatment. Used in filiariasis. May cause impairment of kidney function. Use reserved for cases resistant to less toxic drugs.

Suxamethonium. Muscle relaxant. Acts by depolarization of muscle end plate, rendering the tissue incapable of responding to the neurotransmitter. Action limited by destruction by pseudocholinesterase. Used as an adjunct to anaesthesia for surgery. Short-acting, but effects are prolonged in patients with reduced pseudocholinesterase levels. May cause bradycardia, cardiac arrhythmias, fever, and bronchospasm. Prolonged respiratory paralysis is treated by assisted ventilation and *not* by anticholinesterases.

T

Tacalcitol. Synthetic analogue of CALCITROL (the active form of Vitamin D_3). Inhibits skin cell proliferation without the unwanted effects of calcitrol on calcium balance. Used topically in the treatment of psoriasis. May cause local itching and burning sensation. Calcium balance needs to be monitored if there is pre-existing kidney disease.

Talc. Has lubricant and anti-irritant properties. Used topically on skin and as an aid to the manufacture of some tablets.

Tamoxifen. Antioestrogen. Competes with OESTROGEN for tissue receptor sites. Used as palliative treatment for breast cancer and in treatment of infertility due to failure of ovulation. May cause gastro-intestinal disturbance, fluid retention, hot flushes, and vaginal bleeding.

Tamsulosin. Selective alpha adrenoceptor antagonist with actions on the smooth muscle of the prostate and the lower urinary tract. Used to facilitate micturition/ passing urine when there is an obstruction due to benign prostatic hypertrophy. May cause dizziness, headache, hypotension and abnormal ejaculation.

Tannic acid. Astringent. Precipitates proteins and forms complexes with some heavy metals and alkaloids. May be used topically on skin for minor burns, abrasions or chilblains. Formerly used orally to reduce absorption of some poisons. May cause liver damage, nausea, and vomiting.

Tartrazine. Orange-coloured dye. Used to colour some foods and medicines. May cause hypersensitivity reactions. Shows cross-sensitivity with ACETYLSALICYLIC ACID.

Tazarotene. Retinoid prodrug applied topically to the skin where it is absorbed and converted by skin protease enzymes to form tazarotenic acid. Used in psoriasis where it reduces the excess production of keratin by the skin cells. Unlike other retinoids ETRETINATE or ACITRETIN it does not have systemic effects. May cause local itching, stinging, redness and dry skin.

Teicoplanin. Antibiotic with actions, uses, and adverse effects similar to VANCOMYCIN.

Temazepam (c) (m). Benzodiazepine tranquillizer/hypnotic similar to NITRAZEPAM, but with shorter duration of action and therefore less tendency to impair CNS function on the following day.

Temocillin. Injectable PENICILLIN broad-spectrum antibiotic with activity against penicillin-resistant organisms. Used in severe, life-threatening infections. Adverse effects similar to other PENICILLINS.

Tenoxicam. Non-steroid anti-inflammatory/ analgesic with a long duration of action suitable for once-daily dosing, for use in arthritis. Adverse effects include gastro-intestinal symptoms, oedema, headache, dizziness, skin rash, blood dyscrasias and prolonged bleeding time.

Terazosin. Vasodilator/antihypertensive, with actions, uses, and adverse effects similar to PRAZOSIN. May also be used to reduce symptoms of urinary obstruction caused by benign prostatic hypertrophy.

Terbinafine. Topical and orally active anti-fungal for treating ringworm (Tinea) infections of skin and nails. May cause gastro-intestinal symptoms including irreversible taste loss and liver dysfunction. May also cause skin rashes associated with myalgia and arthralgia. Rarely, may cause serious skin reactions such as toxic epidermal necrosis.

Terbutaline. Beta-adrenoceptor agonist. Actions, uses, and adverse effects as for SALBUTAMOL.

Terebene. Pleasant-smelling oil used to mask unpleasant odours or tastes and as a vapour to relieve nasal decongestion. Large doses are irritant to the gastro-intestinal tract.

Terfenadine. Antihistamine, with actions and adverse effects similar to PROMETHAZINE but is claimed to produce less sedation. Serious cardiac arrhythmias can occur if taken with certain antibiotics, antifungals or grapefruit juice. Contraindicated in patients with cardiac or hepatic disease. Used for hay fever and allergic skin conditions.

Terlipressin. Prodrug which, after injection, is converted in the body into VASOPRESSIN.

Terodiline. Relaxes smooth muscle through several mechanisms, including anticholinergic and calcium antagonist actions. Used to reduce bladder tone in treatment of urinary frequency and incontinence. Adverse effects include dry mouth, blurred vision, constipation, tachycardia and life-threatening ventricular heart arrhythmias.

Testosterone. Male sex hormone. Controls development and maintenance of male sex hormones and secondary sex characteristics (androgenic effects). Also produces metabolic effects that lead to increased growth of bone, water retention, increased production of red blood cells, and increased blood vessel formation in the skin (anabolic effects). Used in the male to speed sexual development, but of no value in treating sterility or impotence unless related to sexual underdevelopment. In the female used to treat some menstrual disorders, for suppression of lactation, and to reduce growth of breast tumours. Has also been used for anabolic effects in debilitated patients, but now superseded by new drugs. Unwanted effects include excess fluid and water retention, stimulation of growth of prostate tumours, and virilization in females. May be administered orally, by injection, implant or transdermal patch.

Tetanus vaccine. Vaccine for prevention of tetanus. Prepared from the tetanus toxin which has been deactivated by chemical treatment.

Tetrabenazine. Used to suppress abnormal movements (e.g., Huntington's chorea). Adverse effects include drowsiness, gastrointestinal upsets, and depression.

Tetracaine. rINN for AMETHOCAINE.

Tetrachloroethylene. Used in treatment of hookworms. Adverse effects include nausea, vomiting, diarrhoea, and vertigo.

Tetracosactide. rINN for TETRACOSACTRIN.

Tetracosactrin. Synthetic polypeptide, with actions, uses, and adverse effects similar to CORTICOTROPHIN. Used intravenously as a test of adrenal function or by depot injection for treatment of inflammatory or degenerative disorders.

Tetracycline. Bacteriostatic antibiotic, active against many gram-positive and gram-negative organisms, some viruses and chlamydia. Adverse effects include diarrhoea and *Candida* bowel superinfection, yellow discolouration of teeth, inhibition of bone growth in children, and exacerbation of renal failure. Interacts in the bowel with compounds of iron, calcium, and aluminium to produce insoluble chelates that are not absorbed.

Thenyldiamine. Antihistamine, with actions, uses, and adverse effects similar to PROMETHAZINE but shorter duration of action.

Theobromine. Xanthine derivative. No useful CNS stimulant effects. Has been used as a diuretic or to dilate coronary or peripheral arteries. Now superseded by more effective agents but still found in some mixtures.

Theophylline. May be used as a bronchodilator, but AMINOPHYLLINE and other derivatives are more commonly used as bronchial muscle relaxants.

Theophylline ethylenediamine. *See* AMINOPHYLLINE.

Thiabendazole. Used in treatment of roundworms. Adverse effects include nausea, drowsiness, and vertigo.

Thiamine. *See* ANEURINE.

Thiazides. A group of related compounds (e.g., BENDROFLUAZIDE), with diuretic effects. They act at the distal convulated tubule of the kidney to reduce reabsorption of salt and water. Moderately potent, but less so than the 'loop diuretics' (e.g., FRUSEMIDE). Active by mouth within one to two hours and a duration of 12–24 hours. May cause hypokalaemia, hyperglycaemia, and hyperuricaemia. Caution in patients with diabetes mellitus and gout. Used in hypertension where they act partly by reducing the peripheral vascular resistance. May cause impotence.

Thiethylperazine. Phenothiazine with actions similar to CHLORPROMAZINE but with little tranquillizing effect. Used as an antiemetic. Given orally, by injection or as suppository. Adverse effects, etc. as for CHLORPROMAZINE.

Thioacetazone. Anti-tuberculous agent, used as a cheap alternative to *para*-AMINOSALICYLIC ACID. May cause gastro-intestinal symptoms, blurred vision, conjunctivitis, and allergic reactions.

Thioguanine. Cytotoxic drug, with actions, uses, and adverse effects similar to MERCAPTOPURINE.

Thiopental. rINN for THIOPENTONE.

Thiopentone sodium. Very short-acting barbiturate used intravenously for anaesthesia of short duration or induction of anaesthesia prior to use of other anaesthetics. Mode of action and adverse effects similar to AMYLOBARBITONE.

Thioridazine. Phenothiazine tranquillizer similar to CHLORPROMAZINE. Used in treatment of psychoses, confusion, and agitation.

Thio-TEPA. Cytotoxic drug used in neoplastic disease. Adverse effects include bone marrow depression.

Thiothixene. Tranquillizer essentially similar to CHLORPROMAZINE.

Thonzylamine. Antihistamine, with actions, uses, and adverse effects similar to PROMETHAZINE but shorter duration of action.

Threitol dimethane sulphonate. Cytotoxic drug used for treatment of ovarian cancer. May cause gastro-intestinal disturbance, bone marrow suppression, and allergic rashes.

Threonine. Essential amino acid.

Thymol. Disinfectant, similar to but less toxic than PHENOL. Used in mouth washes.

Thymoxamine. Alpha$_{1a}$ adrenoceptor antagonist capable of blocking sympathetic nervous activity in the vascular smooth muscle cells of the penis, used by intrapenile (intracavernous) injection prior to intercourse, as a treatment for failure of erection. Slow onset of action mimics normal intercourse. May cause bruising and pain at site of injection. Occasionally causes systemic effects including headache, dizziness, flushes and dry mouth. Rarely may cause prolonged erection and priapism. Also used in peripheral vascular disease.

Thyrotrophin. Pituitary hormone that stimulates production of thyroid hormones. Used in tests of thyroid function.

Thyroxine. Thyroid hormone. Has a stimulating action in general metabolism which is delayed in onset and prolonged (*see* LIOTHYRONINE). Used in treatment of thyroid deficiency. Doses in excess of requirements may cause thyrotoxic symptoms (e.g., rapid pulse, cardiac arrhythmias, diarrhoea, anxiety features, sweating, weight loss, and muscular weakness). Caution if there is pre-existing heart disease.

Tiabendazole. rINN for THIABENDAZOLE.

Tiaprofenic acid. Non-steroid anti-inflammatory/analgesic, with actions, uses, and adverse effects similar to IBUPROFEN.

Tibolone. A steroid with effects which mimic the action of OESTROGEN, androgen and PROGESTERONE. Used to treat menopausal hot flushes caused by deficiency of OESTROGEN and PROGESTERONE and to prevent postmenopausal osteoporosis. Adverse effects include changes in body weight, dizziness, headache, dermatitis, gastro-intestinal disturbances, and increased facial hair growth.

Ticarcillin. Broad-spectrum PENICILLIN injection reserved for the treatment of severe, life-threatening infections. Dosage must be reduced in the presence of severe renal impairment. Adverse effects similar to other PENICILLINS.

Tiludronic acid. Biphosphonate with actions uses and adverse effects similar to ETIDRONATE.

Timolol. Beta-adrenoceptor blocking drug. Uses and adverse effects as for PROPANOLOL, but mainly used by local conjunctival instillation as eyedrops for glaucoma and orally to prevent recurrence of myocardial infarction.

Tinidazole. Antimicrobial used for prevention of postoperative anaerobic and acute gum infections. May cause nausea, vomiting, and bone marrow suppression.

Tinzaparin. Low molecular weight HEPARIN similar to ENOXAPARIN.

Tioconazole. Topical antifungal used to treat fungal infections of the nails. Similar to KETOCONAZOLE. May cause local irritation.

Tioguanine. rINN for THIOGUANINE.

Titanium dioxide. Dermatological treatment. Reduces itching and absorbs ultraviolet rays. Used topically to prevent sunburn and to treat some forms of eczema.

Tizanidine. Centrally acting alpha$_2$ receptor agonist which reduces muscle spasticity without affecting muscle power. Used in patients with spinal injury or disease and in multiple sclerosis. May cause drowsiness, dry mouth, insomnia and hallucinations.

Tobramycin. Antimicrobial. Actions and adverse effects similar to GENTAMICIN.

Tocainide. Cardiac antiarrhythmic drug with actions similar to LIGNOCAINE, but active after oral administration. May cause blood dyscrasias in long-term use. Reserved for acute life-threatening arrhythmias.

Tolazamide. Antidiabetic, with actions, uses, and adverse effects similar to CHLORPROPAMIDE.

Tolazoline. Alpha-adrenoceptor blocking drug with partial agonist activity and smooth muscle relaxant properties. Used in peripheral vascular disease. Side effects include flushing, tachycardia, nausea, and vomiting.

Tolbutamide. Oral antidiabetic drug, with actions, uses, and adverse effects similar to CHLORPROPAMIDE, but excreted more rapidly and thus shorter-acting. Recommended when there is greater danger of hypoglycaemia (e.g., in the elderly).

Tolcapone. Enzyme inhibitor active against catecholamine-O-methyltransferase (COMT). Added to treatment in Parkinson's disease when therapy with LEVODOPA plus CARBIDOPA or BENSERAZIDE no longer provides adequate control e.g. the on-off phenomenon. Helps to stabilize LEVODOPA concentrations in the periphery without causing an unwanted increase. May be associated with movement disorders, insomnia and gastro-intestinal disturbance.

Tolfenamic acid. Non steroidal anti-inflammatory agent with structural similarities to MEFENAMIC ACID. Used in treatment of migraine. Adverse reactions include gastro-intestinal disturbance, skin reactions and bronchospasm. Liver disturbance has been described.

Tolmetin. Non-steroid anti-inflammatory/analgesic, with actions, uses, and adverse effects similar to IBUPROFEN.

Tolnaftate. Antifungal agent used as cream or powder for skin infections.

Tolterodine. Anticholinergic with increased selectivity for bladder muscle receptors used to treat urinary frequency and incontinence. Similar to OXYBUTYNIN but less likely to cause troublesome adverse effects. May cause dry mouth, drowsiness, headache, dry skin and dry eyes.

Tolu. Balsam obtained from trunk of *Myroxylon balsamum.* Used in cough mixtures for expectorant action and flavour.

Topotecan. Cytotoxic used in treatment of advanced (metastatic) ovarian cancer. May cause gastro-intestinal disturbance, hair loss and bone marrow suppression.

Topiramate. Anticonvulsant. Mode of action not fully understood but enhances the activity of the inhibitory neurotransmitter GABA. Used as an adjunct when existing treatment fails to control convulsions. Adverse effects include confusion, unsteadiness and dizziness.

Torasemide. Diuretic. Actions, uses and adverse effects similar to FRUSEMIDE but has a longer duration of action and relative sparing of potassium loss.

Toremifene. Antioestrogen with actions and adverse effects similar to TAMOXIFEN. Used in treatment of advanced (metastatic) breast cancer.

Tragacanth. Laxative. Increases faecal bulk by the same mechanism as METHYLCELLULOSE. Occasionally causes allergic rashes or asthma.

Tramadol. Synthetic opioid used in the treatment of moderate to severe pain. Actions, uses and adverse effects similar to

PETHIDINE but with a low abuse potential. Not a controlled drug.

Tramazoline. Sympathomimetic agent used topically as nasal decongestant. Actions and adverse effects similar to NAPHAZOLINE.

Trandolapril. ACE inhibitor used to treat hypertension. Actions and adverse effects similar to CAPTOPRIL.

Tranexamic acid. Antifibrinolytic agent, used to reverse effects of STREPTOKINASE or other fibrinolytic activity.

Tranylcypromine. Antidepressant. Inhibits monoamine oxidase. Actions and adverse effects similar to PHENELZINE, but less likely to cause hepatitis. Also has AMPHETAMINE-like properties.

Trazodone. Antidepressant. Blocks neuronal uptake of 5-HYDROXYTRYPTAMINE (serotonin). Unlike the tricyclic antidepressants (e.g., AMITRYPTILINE) does not have anticholinergic properties. Thus, tends to be better tolerated in dose and overdose. Adverse effects include gastric discomfort, dry mouth, headache, dizziness, drowsiness, insomnia, and slight hypotension.

Treosulfan. Cytotoxic drug, used in treatment of ovarian cancer. Metabolized by liver to active, epoxide form. Acts by damaging DNA and thus interfering with cell replication. Adverse effects include gastro-intestinal symptoms, skin reactions, hair loss, and bone marrow depression.

Tretinoin. VITAMIN A derivative. Used topically for acne and to reduce photodamage due to excessive exposure to sunlight. Acts by reducing rate of cell turnover and increasing skin thickness. When used topically may cause local skin irritation, peeling and hypo- or hyper-pigmentation. Used in conjunction with chemotherapy in treatment of acute leukaemia.

Triamcinolone. Potent synthetic CORTICOSTEROID, with actions, etc. similar to CORTISONE. Used mainly for topical treatment of certain skin rashes (e.g. eczema). Also used for relief of hay fever symptoms.

Triamterene. Potassium-sparing diuretic similar to AMILORIDE.

Triazolam. Benzodiazepine tranquillizer/hypnotic, with actions, uses, and adverse effects similar to TEMAZEPAM. Licence withdrawn/under review on the grounds that this drug may cause more adverse effects than other benzodiazepines.

Trichloroethylene. Weak inhalational anaesthetic with good analgesic but poor muscle relaxant properties. Used mostly in short surgical procedures (e.g., in obstetrics). May slow the heart and lead to irregular rhythms. Anaesthesia is sometimes followed by nausea, vomiting and headache. When used as a solution in industry, excessive concentrations may depress liver and kidney function. High concentrations may cause acute poisoning with death in coma.

Trichlorofluoromethane. Aerosol propellant/refrigerant. Produces intense cold by its rapid evaporation and thus makes tissues insensitive to pain. Used for relief of muscle pain and spasm.

Triclocarban. Disinfectant used in skin preparations and shampoo for prevention/treatment of certain bacterial and fungal infections. Large doses may cause methaemoglobinaemia.

Triclofos. Hypnotic/sedative. Hydrolyzed in stomach to trichloroethanol and absorbed as such. More palatable and causes less gastric irritation than CHLORAL HYDRATE to which it is otherwise similar.

Triclosan. Antiseptic solution for preoperative hand and skin disinfection.

Triethanolamine. Emulsifying agent used as ear drops to soften wax for removal. May cause localized skin rashes.

Trifluoperazine. Phenothiazine tranquillizer/ antiemetic similar to CHLORPROMAZINE.

Trifluperidol. Butyrophenone tranquillizer, with actions, uses, and adverse effects similar to HALOPERIDOL.

Trihexyphenidyl. rINN for BENZHEXOL.

Tri-iodothyronine. *See* LIOTHYRONINE.

Tri-isopropylphenoxy-polyethoxyethanol. Dispersant/emulsifying agent. Used to stabilize oil-in-water mixtures and to disperse and repel spermatozoa thus preventing conception.

Trilostane. Used to inhibit synthesis of hormones in the adrenal cortex in conditions such as Cushing's syndrome.

Trimeprazine. Phenothiazine similar to CHLORPROMAZINE. Used for antiemetic, sedative, and antipruritic effects. Adverse effects, etc. as for CHLORPROMAZINE.

Trimetaphan. Antihypertensive, with actions and adverse effects similar to HEXAMETHONIUM, but has very brief duration of action. Used for production of controlled hypotension to reduce blood loss during surgery.

Trimethoprim. Antimicrobial. Inhibits conversion of FOLIC ACID to FOLINIC ACID. Combined with SULPHAMETHOXAZOLE in CO-TRIMOXAZOLE. May also be used on its own for prevention of urinary tract infections. Adverse effects include nausea, vomiting, skin rashes, and bone marrow depression.

Trimipramine. Antidepressant, with actions and adverse effects similar to AMITRIPTYLINE.

Triostam. *See* SODIUM ANTIMONYLGLUCONATE.

Tri-potassium di-citrato bismuthate. Bismuth chelate. Used in treatment of peptic ulcer. May cause blackening of the tongue and faeces, constipation, nausea, and vomiting.

Triprolidine. Antihistamine, with actions, uses, and adverse effects similar to PROMETHAZINE.

Triptorelin. Depot intramuscular injection of growth hormone analogue. Suppresses the release of pituitary growth hormone and reduces circulating concentrations of TESTOSTERONE. Used for this effect in the suppression of advanced cancer of the prostate. Adverse effects include hot flushes, decreased libido, feminisation and bone pain.

Tri-sodium edetate. Chelating agent, used intravenously in hypercalcaemia and locally for lime burns in the eye. Exchanges sodium ions for calcium ions. May cause nausea, diarrhoea, cramp, and pain in the limb receiving the infusion. Excessive doses may cause renal damage.

Troglitazone. Orally active anti-diabetic agent which acts to enhance INSULIN action without stimulating its secretion. Used in type II diabetes either as a single agent or in addition to sulphonylureas or INSULIN, may cause gastro-intestinal disturbance but not lactic acidosis.

Tropicamide. Parasympatholytic, used in the eye as a mydriatic and cycloplegic. Actions, etc. similar to ATROPINE SULPHATE, but has rapid onset and short duration of action.

Tropisetron. Anti-emetic, selective 5-HYDROXYTRYPTAMINE antagonist, which blocks peripheral reflexes from relaying messages to the vomiting centre in the brain. Used to prevent nausea and vomiting during cancer chemotherapy. May cause headache, constipation, diarrhoea and dizziness and, rarely, hypersensitivity reactions.

Troxerutin. Vitamin derivative claimed to improve strength and reduce permeability of blood vessels. Used to treat haemorrhoids and venous disorders in the legs.

Tryptophan. Amino acid, essential component of diet. Converted in the body to 5-HYDROXYTRYPTAMINE (serotonin), a neurotransmitter substance that may be depleted in depression. Used in treatment of depression. May cause nausea, drowsiness and may interact with monoamine oxidase inhibitors (e.g., PHENELZINE). Can only be prescribed by hospital specialists.

Tuberculin. Diagnostic agent for tuberculosis. Intradermal injection produces skin reaction in positive cases. May cause skin necrosis in highly sensitive cases.

Tubocurarine. Non-depolarising skeletal muscle relaxant. Blocks passage of impulses at the neuromuscular junction. Used as an adjunct to anaesthesia. May cause fall in blood pressure and paralysis of respiration. NEOSTIGMINE and ATROPINE SULPHATE plus assisted respiration may be used in treatment of toxic effects.

Tulobuterol. An orally active beta-adrenoceptor agonist with bronchodilator activity similar to SALBUTAMOL. Used prophylactically in reversible obstructive airways disease. Adverse effects similar to

SALBUTAMOL include hypokalaemia, tremor and tachycardia.

Turpentine oil. Extract of pine used externally as a rubefacient. May cause rashes and vomiting. Rarely used internally but acts as an evacuant if given rectally.

Tyloxapol. Mucolytic. Administered by inhalation from a nebulizer. Liquefies mucus and aids expectoration where viscid mucus is troublesome (e.g., chronic bronchitis). May cause inflammation of eyelids. If left open, the solution is prone to bacterial infections.

Typhoid vaccine. Vaccine prepared from the polysaccharide of the capsule of Salmonella typhoid (TYPHIM VI) or as an attenuated live strain of that organism (VIVOTIF). The former is given by parenteral injection and may produce fever, headaches, malaise and local soreness. The latter is taken by mouth as a powder in capsule form and is contraindicated in patients whose immunity is suppressed by drugs or by disease.

Tyrothricin. Antimicrobial. Too toxic for systemic use but used for topical treatment of skin, mouth, or ear infections.

U

Undecenoic acid. Antifungal. Applied topically to skin (e.g., in treatment of tinea pedis (athlete's foot)).

Urea. Osmotic diuretic, with actions and uses similar to MANNITOL. May cause gastric irritation with nausea and vomiting. Intravenous use may cause fall in blood pressure and venous thrombosis at site of injection. Largely superseded by MANNITOL and other diuretics. Topically in a cream it is used to reduce excess scaling (ichthyosis) and soften the skin.

Urea hydrogen peroxide. Disinfectant/deodorant used as a source of HYDROGEN PEROXIDE.

Urethane. Cytotoxic drug. Used in treatment of certain neoplastic diseases but largely superseded by newer drugs. May cause gastro-intestinal disturbance and bone marrow depression. Has also mild hypnotic properties and is used as an anaesthetic for small animals.

Urofollitrophin. Follicle-stimulating hormone that stimulates ovulation and spermatogenesis in men, extracted from human post-menopausal urine.

Urofollitropin. rINN for UROFOLLITROPHIN.

Urokinase. Enzyme produced by the kidney and excreted in urine. Like STREPTOKINASE, it activates plasminogen and is used intravenously to break down blood clots in pulmonary embolism. Adverse effects and their treatment similar to STREPTOKINASE.

Ursodeoxycholic acid. Used to aid dissolution of cholesterol gall stones and to treat primary biliary cirrhosis. May produce diarrhoea.

V

Valaciclovir. Pro-drug of ACYCLOVIR with the same actions and adverse effects. Improves the bioavailability and thus improves effectiveness in the treatment of herpes zoster (shingles), herpes simplex and genital herpes.

Valproic acid. Anticonvulsant. *See* SODIUM VALPROATE.

Valsartan. Antihypertensive. Acts by inhibition of angiotensin II receptor and not by ACE inhibition. Used in essential hypertension. May cause excessive tiredness but appears to be well tolerated.

Vancomycin. Antibiotic, used in infections with PENICILLIN-resistant staphylococci and other potentially serious bacteria. Must be given intravenously. Adverse effects include ototoxicity, pain at injection site, rash, nausea and vomiting.

Vasopressin. Posterior pituitary hormone. Has antidiuretic action on kidney and constricts peripheral blood vessels. Used by injection in diagnosis and treatment of diabetes insipidus. May be used to control bleeding from oesophageal varices. May cause pallor, nausea, eructations, cramps, and angina.

Vecuronium. Skeletal muscle relaxant with uses and adverse effects similar to TUBOCURARINE.

Venlafaxine. Antidepressant with novel chemical structure, but actions similar to tricyclic antidepressants (e.g. AMITRIPTYLINE), i.e. it blocks neuronal uptake of the neurotransmitters, noradrenaline and serotonin but has no anticholinergic effects at therapeutic doses. It is less likely, therefore, to cause cardiac effects or convulsions in therapy or overdose.

Verapamil. Used in prevention of angina of effort, hypertension, and in treatment of cardiac dysrhythmias. May cause nausea, dizziness and fall in blood pressure. Contraindicated in heart failure.

Veratrum. Natural product. Reduces sympathetic tone. Was used in hypertension, but seldom now because of adverse effects which include nausea, vomiting, sweats, dizziness, respiratory depression, and abnormal heart rhythms.

Vigabatrin. Anticonvulsant used in treatment of epilepsy not satisfactorily controlled by other drugs. Acts as an analogue of gamma amino-butyric acid (GABA) a neurotransmitter thought to be deficient in epilepsy, and able to stabilise discharges from epileptic foci. May cause drowsiness, dizziness, irritability, headache and memory disturbances. Agitation may occur in children. Severe persistent visual field disturbances have been reported infrequently.

Viloxazine. Antidepressant with some anticonvulsant properties. Unlike the tricyclic antidepressants (e.g., IMIPRAMINE), it is said to have no anticholinergic or sedative properties. Used in treatment of depression, especially when those effects occur from other drugs. May cause nausea and vomiting. If given with PHENYTOIN may induce toxicity due to that drug. No antidote; overdosage treated symptomatically.

Vinblastine. Cytotoxic alkaloid from West Indian periwinkle, used in neoplastic disease. Adverse effects include neuropathy and bone marrow depression.

Vincristine. Cytotoxic, with actions and adverse effects as for VINBLASTINE.

Vindesine. Semisynthetic cytotoxic derived from VINBLASTINE. Has a broader spectrum of antitumour activity than the parent compound and apparently does not share cross-resistance with VINBLASTINE or VINCRISTINE. Used mainly for leukaemia and malignant melanoma. Adverse effects include haematological, neurological, cutaneous, and gastro-intestinal effects.

Vinorelbine. Semi-synthetic vinca alkaloid with actions and adverse effects similar to VINBLASTINE/VINCRISTINE. Used in the treatment of lung and breast cancers, usually in combination with other drugs.

Viomycin. Antibiotic, with actions and adverse effects similar to STREPTOMYCIN.

Viprynium. Used in treatment of threadworms. Adverse effects include red stools, vomiting, and diarrhoea.

Vitamin A. Fat-soluble vitamin present in liver, dairy products, and some vegetables, essential for normal visual function and for maintenance of epithelial surfaces. Overdosage produces mental changes, hyperkeratosis, hypoprothrombinaemia and foetal abnormalities if taken early in pregnancy.

Vitamin B_1. *See* ANEURINE.

Vitamin B_2. *See* RIBOFLAVINE.

Vitamin B_6. *See* PYRIDOXINE.

Vitamin B_7. *See* NICOTINIC ACID.

Vitamin B_{12}. *See* HYDROXOCOBALAMIN.

Vitamin C (Ascorbic acid). Vitamin found in fruit and vegetables, necessary for normal collagen formation. Deficiency causes scurvy with mucosal bleeding and anaemia. High-dose administration in prophylaxis against common cold is controversial. Similarly, although vitamin C influences the formation of haemaglobin and red cell maturation, its addition to haematinics is of questionable value for most patients.

Vitamin D (Calciferol). Group of fat-soluble vitamins found in dairy products and formed in skin exposed to sunlight. Promotes gut absorption of calcium and its mobilization from bone. Deficiency produces rickets and bone softening. Excess produces hypercalcaemia, ectopic calcification, and renal failure.

Vitamin E (Tocopheryl). Vitamin with no clearly defined requirements or deficiency disease in man. Has been suggested as treatment for habitual abortion, cardiovascular disease, and other conditions.

Vitamin K (Menaphthone, Menadiol, Phytomenadione, Acetomenaphthone). Fat-soluble vitamin responsible for formation of prothrombin and other clotting factors. Used to reverse oral anticoagulants and in bleeding diseases including haemorrhagic disease in the new-born. Excessive dosing may produce haemolysis.

W X Y

Warfarin. Coumarin anticoagulant that interferes with synthesis of clotting factors by the liver. May produce allergic reactions. Overdosage produces haemorrhage controlled by VITAMIN K. Potentiated by drugs such as ACETYLSALICYLIC ACID and PHENYLBUTAZONE which displace from protein binding, and reduced by hepatic enzyme inducers, such as barbiturates. Caution if used in liver disease.

Wheat husk. Concentrated extract of non-absorbable fibre content of wheat. Used as bulking agent in treatment of constipation. May cause flatulence and abdominal distension.

Wool fat. Fat/grease recovered from wool. Resembles the secretion from human sebaceous glands in the skin. Mixed with vegetable or soft paraffin oils it produces emollient creams which penetrate the skin and aid drug absorption through the skin. May cause skin sensitization.

Xamoterol. Partial agonist at cardiac beta-adrenoceptors. It therefore stimulates the force and rate of cardiac contraction, but reduces potentially harmful effects of circulating noradrenaline on the heart. It is used to improve cardiac efficiency in patients with mild heart failure. Adverse effects include palpitations, rashes, dizziness and gastro-intestinal symptoms.

Xipamide. Diuretic with potency similar to FRUSEMIDE but slower onset and longer duration of action. Uses and adverse effects similar to BENDROFLUAZIDE.

Xylometazoline. Sympathomimetic, used topically as nasal decongestant. Actions and adverse effects similar to NAPHAZOLINE.

Yohimbine. Plant extract with alpha-adrenoceptor blocking actions. Said to have aphrodisiac properties but not proven.

Z

Zalcitabine. Antiviral drug which prevents replication of the human immunodeficiency virus (HIV) involved in AIDS. Adverse effects include peripheral neuropathy, pancreatitis, gastro-intestinal disorders, rash, pruritus, sweats, and, rarely, liver failure, oesophageal ulcers and anaphylaxis.

Zidovudine. Antiviral drug which prevents replication of retroviruses, including the human immunodeficiency virus (HIV) involved in AIDS. It does not eliminate the infection, and cannot be regarded as a cure. Adverse effects are common and include nausea, abdominal pain, headache, rash, muscle pains, and anaemia. Acts synergistically with LAMIVUDINE and these drugs may be used in combination.

Zinc chloride. Astringent/deodorant. Used in mouth wash and for application to wounds. Caustic in higher concentrations.

Zinc ichthammol. Mixture of ZINC OXIDE and ICHTHAMMOL used for treatment of eczema..

Zinc naphthenate. Used topically for fungal infections of the skin.

Zinc oleate. Topical treatment for eczema. Actions similar to ZINC OXIDE.

Zinc oxide. Dermatological treatment. Has mild astringent, soothing, and protective effects. Used topically in treatment of eczema and excoriated skin.

Zinc powder. *See* ZINC OXIDE.

Zinc salicylate. Dermatological treatment, with actions and uses similar to ZINC OXIDE.

Zinc sulphate. Astringent used topically for skin wounds/ulcers to assist healing. Also included in some eye drops for minor allergic conjunctivitis. Orally it is an emetic, but is not used for this purpose due to toxic effects. In smaller, sustained release doses, it is used for nutritional zinc deficiency. For zinc-deficiency states, a soluble formulation causes less gastro-intestinal disturbance.

Zinc undecenoate. Antifungal used topically for fungal infections of the skin.

Zolmitriptan. Orally active selective serotonin (5-HT) antagonist used in the symptomatic treatment of migraine. Actions and adverse effects similar to SUMATRIPTAN.

Zolpidem. Hypnotic with similar actions and adverse effects to the benzodiazepine hypnotics (e.g. TEMAZEPAM).

Zopiclone. A non-benzodiazepine hypnotic used for short-term treatment of insomnia. May cause a bitter metallic after-taste, minor gastro-intestinal disturbances and drowsiness. Has similar adverse psychiatric reactions to DIAZEPAM.

Zuclopenthixol. Major tranquillizer with actions similar to CHLORPROMAZINE. Used in treatment of schizophrenia. Sedation and hypotension are predictable adverse effects. Extrapyramidal (parkinsonian) symptoms are less frequent than with CHLORPROMAZINE.

PART II

Trade Names

A

AAA. Mouth and Throat Spray. Local anaesthetic/antiseptic for sore throat: *see* BENZOCAINE, CETALKONIUM.

Abidec. Vitamin mixture: *see* ANEURINE, NICOTINAMIDE, PYRIDOXINE, RIBOFLAVINE, VITAMIN A, VITAMIN C, VITAMIN D.

AC Vax. Vaccine for immunisation against meningitis. Contains inactive groups A and C polysaccharide antigens of Neisseria meningitidis. As type B meningitis is more common in the U.K., this vaccine is mainly recommended for travel to places where types A and C are endemic e.g., parts of Africa, South America and India.

Accupro. Antihypertensive: *see* QUINAPRIL.

Accuretic. Antihypertensive: *see* HYDROCHLOROTHIAZIDE, QUINAPRIL.

Accusite (d). Injectable treatment for genital warts which are caused by the human papilloma virus. Combines a cytotoxic with a vasoconstrictor in order to prolong the presence of the former at the treatment site: *see* ADRENALINE, FLUOROURACIL.

Acepril. Antihypertensive: *see* CAPTOPRIL.

Acezide. Antihypertensive combination: *see* CAPTOPRIL, HYDROCHLOROTHIAZIDE.

Achromycin. Anti-infective: *see* TETRACYCLINE.

Aci-Jel. Jelly for topical treatment of vaginal infection.

Acnecide. Topical gel treatment for acne: *see* BENZOYL PEROXIDE.

Acnegel (d). Topical gel for treatment of acne: *see* BENZOYL PEROXIDE.

Acnidazil. Topical cream for treatment of acne: *see* BENZOYL PEROXIDE, MICONAZOLE.

Actal. Antacid: *see* ALEXITOL SODIUM.

Act-HIB (d). Vaccine: *see* HAEMOPHILUS INFLUENZA TYPE B VACCINE.

Actifed. Decongestant: *see* PSEUDOEPHEDRINE, TRIPROLIDINE.

Actifed Compound Linctus. As Actifed plus DEXTROMETHORPHAN for cough suppression.

Actifed Expectorant. As Actifed with GUAIPHENESIN.

Actilyse. Fibrinolytic: *see* ALTEPLASE.

Actinac. Topical treatment for acne: *see* ALLANTOIN, BUTOXYETHYL NICOTINATE, CHLORAMPHENICOL, HYDROCORTISONE, SULPHUR.

Actonorm. Antacid: *see* ALUMINIUM HYDROXIDE, MAGNESIUM HYDROXIDE, ACTIVATED DIMETHICONE.

Actrapid. Synthetic human crystalline insulin: *see* INSULIN.

Acular. Non steroidal anti-inflammatory used to reduce pain and inflammation after eye surgery: *see* KETOROLAC.

Acupan. Analgesic: *see* NEFOPAM.

Adalat. Antianginal: *see* NIFEDIPINE.

Adalat LA. Controlled-release antianginal antihypertensive: *see* NIFEDIPINE.

Adalat retard. Sustained-release vasodilator antihypertensive: *see* NIFEDIPINE.

Adcortyl. Corticosteroid for topical or systemic use: *see* TRIAMCINOLONE.

Addamel. Electrolytes and trace elements for parenteral nutrition.

Addiphos. Source of phosphate during parenteral feeding.

Adenocor. Antiarrhythmic: *see* ADENOSINE.

Adifax (d). Anti-obesity: *see* DEXFENFLURAMINE.

Adizem-XL/Adizem SR. Controlled release antianginal/antihypertensive: *see* DILTIAZEM.

Adriamycin. Cytotoxic antibiotic: *see* DOXORUBICIN.

Aerocrom. For asthma: *see* SODIUM CROMOGLYCATE.

Aerolin. Sympathomimetic bronchodilator: *see* SALBUTAMOL.

Agarol. Laxative: *see* AGAR, LIQUID PARAFFIN, PHENOLPHTHALEIN.

Aglutella Gentili (b). GLUTEN-free pasta, low in protein, sodium, and potassium. Dietary substitute used in chronic renal failure and phenylketonuria.

Akineton. Anticholinergic, antiparkinsonian: *see* BIPERIDEN.

Alcobon. Antifungal for systemic yeast infections: *see* FLUCYTOSINE.

Alcoderm. Emollient cream/lotion for protection of dry skin: *see* CETYL ALCOHOL, ETHANOLAMINE, LIQUID PARAFFIN, POLYSORBATE 60, SODIUM LAURYL SULPHATE, STEARYL ALCOHOL.

Aldactide. Diuretic/antihypertensive: *see* HYDROFLUMETHIAZIDE, SPIRONOLACTONE.

Aldactone. Diuretic: *see* SPIRONOLACTONE.

Aldomet. Antihypertensive: *see* METHYLDOPA.

Alec. For treatment of infantile respiratory distress syndrome: *see* PUMACTANT.

Alembicol D (b). Lipid extract of coconut oil; substitute for long-chain fats in fat malabsorption.

Alfazine. Nasal decongestant: *see* OXYMETAZOLINE.

Algesal. Rubefacient: *see* DIETHYLAMINE SALICYLATE.

Algicon. Antacid: *see* ALUMINIUM HYDROXIDE, MAGNESIUM ALGINATE, MAGNESIUM CARBONATE, POTASSIUM BICARBONATE.

Algipan. Rubefacient: *see* CAPSICUM, NICOTINIC ACID, SALICYLIC ACID.

Algitec. Antacid/gastric histamine receptor blocker to reduce gastro-oesophageal reflux: *see* ALGINIC ACID, CIMETIDINE.

Alimix (d). For treatment of gastric reflux and delayed gastric emptying: *see* CISAPRIDE.

Alka-Donna. Antacid: *see* ALUMINIUM HYDROXIDE, BELLADONNA EXTRACT, MAGNESIUM TRISILICATE.

Alkeran. Cytotoxic: *see* MELPHALAN.

Allegron. Antidepressant: *see* NORTRIPTYLINE.

Almazine. Anxiolytic: *see* LORAZEPAM.

Almevax. Live attenuated RUBELLA VACCINE.

Alomide. Anti-allergic for allergic conjunctivitis: *see* LODOXAMIDE.

Alophen. Purgative: *see* ALOIN, BELLADONNA EXTRACT, IPECACUANHA, PHENOLPHTHALEIN.

Alphaderm. Topical corticosteroid cream: *see* HYDROCORTISONE, UREA.

Alphagan. Eye-drops for treatment of glaucoma: *see* BRIMONIDINE.

Alphaglobin. For primary and secondary antibody deficiency disorders and idiopathic thrombocytopenic purpura: *see* IMMUNOGLOBULIN.

Alpha Keri Bath. Emollient bath additive for dry skin: *see* LIQUID PARAFFIN, WOOL FAT.

Alphaparin. Anticoagulant for prevention of postoperative thromboembolism: *see* CERTOPARIN.

Alphosyl. Topical treatments for psoriasis and other scaly disorders: *see* ALLANTOIN, COAL TAR.

Alphosyl HC. Topical steroid treatment for psoriasis: *see* ALLANTOIN, COAL TAR, HYDROCORTISONE.

Altacite. Antacid: *see* HYDROTALCITE.

Alu-Cap. Antacid: *see* ALUMINIUM HYDROXIDE.

Aludrox. Antacid: *see* ALUMINIUM HYDROXIDE.

Aludrox SA. Antacid/sedative: *see* ALUMINIUM HYDROXIDE, AMBUTONIUM, MAGNESIUM HYDROXIDE.

Aluline. For gout: *see* ALLOPURINOL.

Alunex. Anti-allergic: *see* CHLORPHENIRAMINE.

Alupent. Sympathomimetic bronchodilator: *see* ORCIPRENALINE.

Alupram. Anxiolytic: *see* DIAZEPAM.

Aluzine. Diuretic: *see* FRUSEMIDE.

Alvedon. Analgesic/antipyretic suppository: *see* PARACETAMOL.

Alvercol. Antispasmodic/laxative for treatment of irritable bowel syndrome and other causes of increased muscle spasms in the large bowel: *see* STERCULIA, ALVERINE.

Ambisome. Antifungal: *see* AMPHOTERICIN.

Ametop. Anaesthetic gel for use prior to taking a blood sample (venepuncture): *see* AMETHOCAINE.

Amias. Antihypertensive: *see* CANDESARTAN CILEXETIL.

Amikin. Antibiotic: *see* AMIKACIN.

Amilco. Diuretic combination: *see* AMILORIDE, HYDROCHLOROTHIAZIDE.

Aminogran (b). Low AMINO ACIDS food substitute for phenylketonuria.

Aminoplasmal. Intravenous AMINO ACIDS and electrolytes for parenteral nutrition.

Aminoplex 5 and 14. Intravenous AMINO ACIDS, SORBITOL, MALIC ACID, VITAMINS and electrolytes.

Amoxil. Antibiotic: *see* AMOXYCILLIN.

Amphocil. Antifungal: *see* AMPHOTERICIN.

Ampiclox. Antibiotic: *see* AMPICILLIN, CLOXACILLIN.

Amsidine. Cytotoxic: *see* AMSACRINE.

Amytal (c). Hypnotic/minor tranquillizer: *see* AMYLOBARBITONE.

Anabact. Topical antibacterial: *see* METRONIDAZOLE.

Anacal. Topical treatment for haemorrhoids: *see* HEXACHLOROPHANE, PREDNISOLONE, HEPARINOID.

Anaflex lozenges. Antiseptic for mouth and throat: *see* POLYNOXYLIN.

Anaflex topical preps. Skin antiseptic: *see* POLYNOXYLIN.

Anafranil. Antidepressant: *see* CLOMIPRAMINE.

Analog (b). Range of oral dietary supplements for management of inherited metabolic disorders in infants.

Androcur. For male sexual disorders: *see* CYPROTERONE.

Andropatch. Transdermal patch for male sex hormone replacement therapy in both primary or secondary deficiency: *see* TESTOSTERONE.

Anectine. Muscle relaxant during anaesthesia: *see* SUXAMETHONIUM.

Anexate. Benzodiazepine antagonist: *see* FLUMAZENIL.

Angettes. Enteric-coated aspirin to reduce the risk of thrombosis: *see* ACETYLSALICYLIC ACID.

Angilol. Beta-adrenoceptor blocker: *see* PROPRANOLOL.

Angiopine MR. Sustained release antianginal, antihypertensive: *see* NIFEDIPINE.

Anhydrol forte. Antiperspirant: *see* ALUMINIUM CHLORIDE.

Anodesyn. Local treatment for haemorrhoids: *see* ALLANTOIN, BRONOPOL, EPHEDRINE, LIGNOCAINE.

Anquil. Tranquillizer: *see* BENPERIDOL.

Antabuse. For treatment of alcoholism: *see* DISULFIRAM.

Antepar. For threadworms and roundworms: *see* PIPERAZINE.

Antepsin. Mucosal protective for treatment of peptic ulceration: *see* SUCRALFATE.

Antoin. Analgesic: *see* ACETYLSALICYLIC ACID, CAFFEINE, CODEINE.

Anturan. Increases urate excretion in gout: *see* SULPHINPYRAZONE.

Anugesic-HC. Topical treatment for haemorrhoids: *see* BENZYL, BENZOATE, HYDROCORTISONE, PRAMOXINE, ZINC OXIDE, BISMUTH OXIDE, BISMUTH SUBGALLATE.

Anusol. Local treatment for haemorrhoids: *see* BISMUTH BENZOATE, BISMUTH SUBGALLATE, BISMUTH OXIDE, ZINC OXIDE.

Anusol HC. As Anusol plus HYDROCORTISONE.

Apresoline. Antihypertensive: *see* HYDRALAZINE.

Aprinox. Diuretic: *see* BENDROFLUAZIDE.

Aproten (b). GLUTEN-free products for coeliac disease.

Aprovel. Antihypertensive: *see* IRBESARTAN

Apsifen. Non-steroid anti-inflammatory/ analgesic: *see* IBUPROFEN.

Apsin V.K. Antibiotic: *see* PHENOXYMETHYLPENICILLIN.

Apsolol. Beta-adrenoceptor blocker: *see* PROPRANOLOL.

Apsolox. Beta-adrenoceptor blocker: *see* OXPRENOLOL.

Aquadrate. Keratolytic for thickened, dry skin: *see* UREA.

Aramine. Vasoconstrictor for shock: *see* METARAMINOL.

Aredia. For treatment of tumour-induced hypercalcaemia, Paget's disease, osteolytic lesions, and bone pain associated with multiple myeloma and breast cancer: *see* PAMIDRONATE.

Arelix (d). Diuretic: *see* PIRETANIDE.

Arfonad. Hypotensive: *see* TRIMETAPHAN.

Aricept. To improve symptoms of mild or moderate Alzheimer's disease: *see* DONEPEZIL.

Arilvax. Vaccine for immunization against yellow fever.

Arimidex. Anti-oestrogen for treating advanced breast cancer in post-menopausal women: *see* ANASTROZOLE.

Arpicolin. Syrup formulation. Anticholinergic/antiparkinsonian: *see* PROCYCLIDINE.

Arpimycin. Antibiotic: *see* ERYTHROMYCIN.

Arret. Antidiarrhoeal: *see* LOPERAMIDE.

Arthrotec. Anti-inflammatory with prostaglandin analogue for protection against ulceration of the stomach: *see* DICLOFENAC, MISOPROSTOL.

Artracin. Non-steroid anti-inflammatory/analgesic: *see* INDOMETHACIN.

Arvin (d). Anticoagulant: *see* ANCROD.

Arythmol. Antiarrhythmic for treatment and prophylaxis of ventricular arrhythmias: *see* PROPAFENONE.

Asacol. For ulcerative colitis: *see* MESALAZINE.

Ascabiol. Topical treatment for scabies and lice: *see* BENZYL BENZOATE.

Asendis. Tricyclic antidepressant: *see* AMOXAPINE.

Aserbine. Desloughing cream/solution for removal of clots and slough in wounds or ulcers: *see* BENZOIC ACID, MALIC ACID, PROPYLENE GLYCOL, SALICYLIC ACID.

Asilone. Antacid: *see* ALUMINIUM HYDROXIDE, DIMETHICONE, MAGNESIUM OXIDE

Asmabec. Steroid aerosol for asthma: *see* BECLOMETHASONE

Asmasal. Sympathomimetic bronchodilator aerosol: *see* SALBUTAMOL

Asmaven. Sympathomimetic bronchodilator: *see* SALBUTAMOL.

Aspav. Water-dispersable, analgesic tablets: *see* ACETYLSALICYLIC ACID, PAPAVERETUM.

A.T. 10. For Vitamin D deficiency or resistance: *see* DIHYDROTACHYSTEROL.

Atarax. Sedative/tranquillizer: *see* HYDROXYZINE.

Atensine. Sedative/tranquillizer: *see* DIAZEPAM.

Ativan. Sedative/tranquillizer: *see* LORAZEPAM.

Atromid-S 500. Antianginal/lipid-lowering agent: *see* CLOFIBRATE.

Atrovent. Bronchodilator for inhalation: *see* IPRATROPIUM.

Attenuvax. Live attenuated MEASLES VACCINE with NEOMYCIN as antibiotic preservative.

Audax. Drops for middle and outer ear infection: *see* CHOLINE SALICYLATE.

Audicort. Drops for outer ear infection: *see* BENZOCAINE, NEOMYCIN, TRIAMCINOLONE, UNDECENOIC ACID.

Audinorm. Drops for removal of ear wax: *see* GLYCERIN, DOCUSATE SODIUM.

Augmentin. Antibacterial: *see* AMOXYCILLIN, CLAVULANIC ACID.

Auraltone. Drops for middle ear pain: *see* BENZOCAINE, PHENAZONE.

Aureocort. Topical treatment for allergic/infective skin conditions: *see* CHLORTETRACYCLINE, TRIAMCINOLONE.

Aureomycin. Antibiotic: *see* CHLORTETRACYCLINE.

Aveeno. For addition to bath for skin allergy.

Avloclor. Antimalarial: *see* CHLOROQUINE.

Avomine. Antihistamine/antiemetic: *see* PROMETHAZINE.

Axid. Gastric histamine receptor blocker; reduces acid secretion: *see* NIZATIDINE.

Axsain. Topical treatment for post-herpetic neuralgia (pain persisting after resolution of shingles) and relief of painful diabetic neuropathy: *see* CAPSAICIN.

Azactam. Antibiotic: *see* AZTREONAM.

Azamune (d). Cytotoxic: *see* AZATHIOPRINE.

B

Bactigras. Impregnated wound dressing: *see* CHLORHEXIDINE.

Bactrim (d). Antibacterial: *see* CO-TRIMOXAZOLE.

Bactroban. Topical antibiotic: *see* MUPIROCIN.

Balmosa. Rubefacient: *see* METHYL SALICYLATE, MENTHOL, CAMPHOR, CAPSICUM.

Balneum. Topical application for dry skin: *see* SOYA OIL, COAL TAR.

Baltar. Shampoo for psoriasis and eczema of the scalp: *see* COAL TAR.

Bambec. Bronchodilator: *see* BAMBUTEROL.

Baratol. Antihypertensive: *see* INDORAMIN.

Baxan. Antibiotic: *see* CEFADROXIL.

Baycaron. Diuretic: *see* MEFRUSIDE.

B.C. 500. Vitamin mixture: *see* ANEURINE, CYANOCOBALAMIN, NICOTINAMIDE, PYRIDOXINE, RIBOFLAVINE, VITAMIN C, CALCIUM PANTOTHENATE.

Beclazone. Steroid aerosol for asthma: *see* BECLOMETHASONE.

Becloforte. Steroid aerosol for asthma: *see* BECLOMETHASONE.

Becodisks. Inhalation system for treatment of asthma: *see* BECLOMETHASONE.

Beconase. Nasal aerosol for allergic rhinitis: *see* BECLOMETHASONE.

Becosym. Vitamin B complex: *see* ANEURINE, NICOTINAMIDE, PYRIDOXINE, RIBOFLAVINE.

Becotide. Steroid aerosol for asthma: *see* BECLOMETHASONE.

Bedranol. Beta-adrenoceptor blocker: *see* PROPRANOLOL.

Bellocarb. For reducing gastro-intestinal motility and secretion: *see* BELLADONNA EXTRACT, MAGNESIUM TRISILICATE, MAGNESIUM CARBONATE.

Benadon. Antiemetic: *see* PYRIDOXINE.

Bendogen. Antihypertensive: *see* BETHANIDINE.

Benemid. Uricosuric for gout: *see* PROBENECID.

Benerva. Vitamin B_1 for deficiency: *see* ANEURINE.

Benerva compound. Vitamin B mixture for deficiency: *see* ANEURINE, NICOTINAMIDE, RIBOFLAVINE.

Bengue's balsam. Rubefacient: *see* METHYL SALICYLATE.

Benoral. Non-steroid anti-inflammatory/analgesic: *see* BENORYLATE.

Benoxyl. Topical treatment for acne: *see* BENZOYL PEROXIDE.

Bentex. Antiparkinsonian: *see* BENZHEXOL.

Benylin Chesty Cough. Cough suppressant: *see* DIPHENHYDRAMINE, MENTHOL.

Benylin with codeine. As Benylin Chesty Cough with CODEINE.

Benylin Mentholated. As Benylin Chesty Cough with DEXTROMETHORPHAN, PSEUDOEPHEDRINE.

Benzamycin. Tropical treatment for acne: *see* BENZOYL PEROXIDE, ERYTHROMYCIN.

Berkatens. For treatment of angina, hypertension and arrhythmias: *see* VERAPAMIL.

Berkmycen. Antibiotic: *see* OXYTETRACYCLINE.

Berkolol. Beta-adrenoceptor blocker: *see* PROPRANOLOL.

Berkozide. Diuretic: *see* BENDROFLUAZIDE.

Berotec. Bronchodilator for asthma: *see* FENOTEROL.

Beta-Adalat. Antihypertensive: *see* ATENOLOL, NIFEDIPINE.

Betacap. Topical treatment for scalp psoriasis: *see* BETAMETHASONE.

Beta-Cardone. Beta-adrenoceptor blocker: *see* SOTALOL.

Betadine. Antiseptic: *see* PROVIDONE-IODINE.

Betaferon. For reduction of frequency and severity of relapses in multiple sclerosis: *see* INTERFERON BETA-1B.

Betagan. Beta-adrenoceptor blocker eye drops for treatment of glaucoma: *see* LEVOBUNOLOL.

Betaloc. Beta-adrenoceptor blocker: *see* METOPROLOL.

Beta-Prograne. Sustained-release antihypertensive: *see* PROPRANOLOL.

Betim. Beta-adrenoceptor blocker: *see* TIMOLOL.

Betnelan. Corticosteroid: *see* BETAMETHASONE.

Betnesol. Soluble corticosteroid tablets and injection: *see* BETAMETHASONE.

Betnesol-N. Topical corticosteroid/ antibiotic: *see* BETAMETHASONE, NEOMYCIN.

Betnovate. Topical corticosteroid: *see* BETAMETHASONE.

Betnovate C. Topical corticosteroid/ anti-infective: *see* BETAMETHASONE, CLIOQUINOL.

Betnovate N. Topical corticosteroid/ antibiotic: *see* BETAMETHASONE, NEOMYCIN.

Betnovate Rectal. Topical corticosteroid for haemorrhoids: *see* BETAMETHASONE, LIGNOCAINE, PHENYLEPHRINE.

Betoptic. Eye drops for glaucoma: *see* BETAXOLOL.

Bezalip. Lipid-lowering agent: *see* BEZAFIBRATE.

Bi-Aglut (b). GLUTEN-free biscuits for gluten-sensitive bowel disorders.

Bicillin. Antibiotic: *see* BENZYLPENICILLIN, PROCAINE PENICILLIN.

BICNU. Cytotoxic: *see* CARMUSTINE.

Bilarcil. Antischistosomiasis: *see* METRIPHONATE.

Biltricide. Antischistosomiasis: *see* PRAZIQUANTEL.

BiNovum. Oral contraceptive: *see* ETHINYLOESTRADIOL, NORETHISTERONE.

Bioplex. Mouthwash for treatment of oral aphthous ulcers: *see* CARBENOXOLONE.

Bioral. Topical therapy for mouth ulcers: *see* CARBENOXOLONE.

Biorphen. Anticholinergic/ antiparkinsonian: *see* ORPHENADRINE.

Bismodyne. Cream for topical application to relieve pain and irritation from haemorrhoids and other causes of anal discomfort: *see* BISMUTH SUBGALLATE, HEXACHLOROPHANE, LIGNOCAINE, ZINC OXIDE.

Blocadren. Beta-adrenoceptor blocker: *see* TIMOLOL.

Bocasan. Antiseptic mouthwash for oral infections: *see* SODIUM PERBORATE.

Bonefos. For treatment of hypercalcaemia induced by malignant disease: *see* SODIUM CLODRONATE.

Bonjela. Topical therapy for mouth ulcers: *see* CETALKONIUM, CHOLINE SALICYLATE.

Botox. To treat spasms of muscles of the face and eye: *see* BOTULINUM TOXIN.

Bradosol. Antiseptic for mouth and throat infections: *see* DOMIPHEN.

Brasivol. Topical abrasive/cleansing paste for acne: *see* ALUMINIUM OXIDE.

Bretylate. Antiarrhythmic: *see* BRETYLIUM.

Brevinor. Oral contraceptive: *see* ETHINYLOESTRADIOL, NORETHISTERONE.

Bricanyl. Sympathomimetic bronchodilator: *see* TERBUTALINE.

Brietal Sodium. Short-acting barbiturate for short-duration anaesthesia: *see* METHOHEXITONE.

Britaject. Antiparkinsonian: *see* APOMORPHINE.

Britiazim (d). Antianginal: *see* DILTIAZEM.

Britlofex. For relief of symptoms during withdrawal from opiate addiction: *see* LOFEXIDINE.

Brocadopa Temtabs (d). Sustained-release formulation of Brocadopa.

Broflex. Antiparkinsonian/anticholinergic: *see* BENZHEXOL.

Brolene ophthalmic preps. Anti-infective drops/ointment for use in the eye: *see* PROPAMIDINE.

Bronchodil. Sympathetic bronchodilator: *see* REPROTEROL.

Brufen. Non-steroid anti-inflammatory/ analgesic: *see* IBUPROFEN.

Brulidine. Topical anti-infective for burns, wounds: *see* DIBROMOPROPAMIDINE.

Buccastem. Anti-emetic tablet for buccal absorption: *see* PROCHLORPERAZINE.

Burinex. Diuretic: *see* BUMETANIDE.

Burinex A. Diuretic: *see* AMILORIDE, BUMETANIDE.

Burinex K. As Burinex plus POTASSIUM CHLORIDE supplement.

Buscopan. Anticholinergic/antispasmodic for gastro-intestinal or uterine spasm: *see* HYOSCINE BUTYLBROMIDE.

Buspar. Anxiolytic: *see* BUSPIRONE.

Butacote. Non-steroid anti-inflammatory/analgesic: *see* PHENYLBUTAZONE. Enteric-coated to reduce gastric irritation.

C

Cabaser. To control symptoms of Parkinson's disease: *see* CABERGOLINE.

Cacit. Effervescent calcium supplement for treatment of deficiency states and osteoporosis: *see* CALCIUM CARBONATE, CALCIUM CITRATE.

Cacit D3. For vitamin and calcium deficiency, or for osteoporosis: *see* CALCIUM CITRATE, VITAMIN D3.

Cafergot. Vasoconstrictor for migraine: *see* CAFFEINE, ERGOTAMINE.

Calaband. Impregnated bandage for dressing skin wounds and ulcers: *see* BORIC ACID, CALAMINE, CASTOR OIL, GLYCERIN, ZINC OXIDE.

Caladryl. Cream or lotion for skin irritation (e.g., sunburn, insect bites): *see* CALAMINE, DIPHENHYDRAMINE, CAMPHOR.

Calceos. For vitamin and calcium deficiency, or for osteoporosis: *see* CALCIUM, VITAMIN D3.

Calcichew. Antacid: *see* CALCIUM CARBONATE.

Calcichew D3. Calcium supplement with vitamin D3 for treatment of deficiency states, osteoporosis, and osteomalacia: *see* CALCIUM CHOLECALCIFEROL.

Calcijex. Vitamin for intravenous administration in patients with chronic renal failure: *see* CALCITRIOL.

Calcimax. Calcium/vitamin supplements for calcium deficiencies: *see* ANEURINE, NICOTINIC ACID, PANTOTHENIC ACID, PYRIDOXINE, RIBOFLAVINE, VITAMIN C, CALCIUM LAEVULINATE, CALCIUM CHLORIDE.

Calciparine. Anticoagulant: *see* HEPARIN.

Calcisorb. For prevention of hypercalcuria and renal stones: *see* SODIUM CELLULOSE PHOSPHATE.

Calcitare. Hormone: *see* CALCITONIN.

Calcium heparin. Anticoagulant: *see* HEPARIN.

Calcium leucovorin. Antagonizes antifolate cytotoxic drugs: *see* FOLINIC ACID.

Calcium Resonium. Ion exchange resin: *see* CALCIUM POLYSTYRENE SULPHONATE.

Calcium-Sandoz. Calcium supplement for deficiency (e.g., tetany).

Calmurid. Keratolytic cream for removal of dry, scaly skin: *see* UREA, LACTIC ACID.

Calmurid HC. Corticosteroid cream for eczema: *see* HYDROCORTISONE, UREA, LACTIC ACID.

Calogen (b). Contains arachis oil, a source of high energy for use in renal failure.

Caloreen (b). Protein-free, high-calorie powder for use when low-protein diet is needed (e.g., kidney failure).

Calpol. Analgesic elixir: *see* PARACETAMOL.

Calsynar. Hormone: *see* CALCITONIN.

C.A.M. Bronchodilator elixir for children: *see* BUTETHAMATE, EPHEDRINE.

Camcolit. Antidepressant for manic depressive psychosis: *see* LITHIUM SALTS.

Campral EC. A synthetic GABA analogue for maintaining abstinence after alcohol withdrawal: *see* ACAMPROSATE.

Campto. Cytotoxic: *see* IRINOTECAN.

Canesten. Antifungal: *see* CLOTRIMAZOLE.

Canesten HC. Topical anti-infective/ corticosteroid. As Canestan plus HYDROCORTISONE.

Capasal. Shampoo for dry and scaly scalp conditions: *see* COAL TAR, SALICYLIC ACID.

Capastat. Anti-tuberculous antibiotic: *see* CAPREOMYCIN.

Caplenal. For gout: *see* ALLOPURINOL.

Capoten. Antihypertensive: *see* CAPTOPRIL.

Capozide. Antihypertensive combination: *see* CAPTOPRIL, HYDROCHLOROTHIAZIDE.

Caprin. Slow-release analgesic: *see* ACETYLSALICYLIC ACID.

Carace. Antihypertensive: *see* LISINOPRIL.

Carace plus. Antihypertensive: *see* HYDROCHLOROTHIAZIDE, LISINOPRIL.

Carbalax. Phosphate enema: *see* SODIUM ACID PHOSPHATE.

Carbellon. Antacid/sedative: *see* BELLADONNA EXTRACT, CHARCOAL, MAGNESIUM HYDROXIDE, PEPPERMINT OIL.

Carbo-Cort (d). Corticosteroid cream for eczema and other skin rashes: *see* COAL TAR, HYDROCORTISONE.

Carbo-Dome. Topical treatment for psoriasis: *see* COAL TAR.

Carbomix. Oral adsorbant for treatment of acute poisoning and drug overdose: *see* ACTIVATED CHARCOAL.

Cardene. Antianginal, antihypertensive: *see* NICARDIPINE.

Cardene SR. Sustained release antianginal, antihypertensive: *see* NICARDIPINE.

Cardilate MR. Antihypertensive, antianginal: *see* NIFEDIPINE.

Cardura. Antihypertensive: *see* DOXAZOSIN.

Carisoma. Muscle relaxant: *see* CARISOPRODOL.

Carobel. Carob seed flour for thickening feeds in the treatment of vomiting.

Carylderm. Insecticide lotion shampoo for treatment of lice: *see* CARBARYL.

Casilan (b). High-protein, low-salt food for hypoproteinaemia.

Casodex. Antiandrogen used in treatment of carcinoma of the prostate gland: *see* BICALUTAMIDE.

Catapres. Antihypertensive: *see* CLONIDINE.

Caverject. Prostaglandin injection for intracavernous (penile) injection in treatment of erectile dysfunction: *see* ALPROSTADIL.

Ceanel (b). Shampoo for psoriasis: *see* CETRIMIDE, UNDECENOIC ACID.

Cedax. Antibiotic: *see* CEFTIBUTEN.

Cedocard. Antianginal: *see* ISOSORBIDE NITRATE.

Cefrom. Cephalosporin antibiotic: *see* CEFPIROME.

Celance. Antiparkinsonian: *see* PERGOLIDE.

Celbenin. Antibiotic: *see* METHICILLIN.

Celectol. Antihypertensive: *see* CELIPROLOL.

Celevac. Purgative: *see* METHYLCELLULOSE.

Cellcept. Immunosuppressant for prevention of rejection of kidney transplants: *see* MYCOPHENOLATE.

Ceporex. Antibiotic: *see* CEPHALEXIN.

Cernevit. Parenteral vitamin supplement: *see* BIOTIN, CHOLECALCIFEROL, CYANOCOBALAMIN, FOLIC ACID, GLYCINE, NICOTINAMIDE, PANTOTHENIC ACID, PYRIDOXINE, RIBOFLAVINE, THIAMINE, VITAMIN A, VITAMIN C, VITAMIN E.

Cerumol. Drops for removal of ear wax: *see* CHLORBUTOL, PARADICHLOROBENZENE, ARACHIS OIL.

Cervagem. Pessary for use prior to surgical termination of pregnancy: *see* GEMEPROST.

Cesamet. Antiemetic: *see* NABILONE.

Cetavlex. Topical anti-infective for minor abrasions: *see* CETRIMIDE.

Chemotrim. Antibacterial: *see* CO-TRIMOXAZOLE.

Chendol (d). Bile acid for dissolution of cholesterol gall stones: *see* CHENODEOXYCHOLIC ACID.

Chenofalk. Bile acid for dissolution of cholesterol gall stones: *see* CHENODEOXYCHOLIC ACID.

Chimax. Sex hormone for treatment of prostatic carcinoma: *see* FLUTAMIDE.

Chlorasol. Solution for cleansing and desloughing of skin ulcers: *see* SODIUM HYPOCHLORITE.

Chocovite. For calcium deficiency: *see* CALCIUM GLUCONATE, VITAMIN D.

Choledyl (d). Bronchodilator: *see* CHOLINE THEOPHYLLINATE.

Choragon. Hormone: *see* GONADOTROPHIN.

Cicatrin. Topical anti-infective: *see* BACITRACIN, CYSTEINE, GLYCINE, NEOMYCIN, THREONINE.

Cidomycin. Antibiotic for injection or topical use: *see* GENTAMICIN.

Cilest. Oral contraceptive: *see* ETHINYLOESTRADIOL, NORGESTIMATE.

Ciloxan. Antibiotic for treatment of eye infections: *see* CIPROFLOXACIN.

Cinobac. Antibacterial: *see* CINOXACIN.

Cipramil. Antidepressant: *see* CITALOPRAM.

Ciproxin. Antibiotic: *see* CIPROFLOXACIN.

Citanest. Local anaesthetic for minor surgery: *see* PRILOCAINE.

Citanest with Octapressin. As Citanest plus vasoconstrictor to prolong action: *see* FELYPRESSIN.

Citramag. Purgative for use prior to surgery: *see* MAGNESIUM CITRATE.

Citrical. Oral calcium supplement for deficiency: *see* CALCIUM CARBONATE.

Claforan. Antibiotic: *see* CEFOTAXIME.

Clairvan. Respiratory stimulant: *see* ETHAMIVAN.

Clarityn. Antihistamine: *see* LORATADINE.

Clexane. Anticoagulant to reduce the risk of thrombosis after surgery: *see* ENOXAPARIN.

Climagest. Hormone replacement therapy for treatment of menopausal symptoms: *see* OESTRADIOL, NORETHISTERONE.

Climaval. Hormone replacement therapy for relief of menopausal symptoms after hysterectomy: *see* OESTRADIOL.

Climesse. Sex hormone for post-menopausal symptoms and prophylaxis of post-menopausal osteoporosis: *see* NORETHISTERONE, OESTRADIOL.

Clinifeed (b). Liquid feeds for enteral absorption. Given via naso-gastric tube or enterostomy as treatment or prevention of malnourishment (e.g., postoperatively).

Clinitar. Cream and shampoo for psoriasis and eczema: *see* COAL TAR.

Clinoril. Non-steroid anti-inflammatory/analgesic: *see* SULINDAC.

Cloburate. Corticosteroid eye drops: cream or ointment for skin: *see* CLOBETASONE.

Clomid. Sex hormone: *see* CLOMIPHENE.

Clopixol. Major tranquillizer administered as long-acting injection: *see* ZUCLOPENTHIXOL.

Clostet. Tetanus vaccine.

Clotam. A non steroidal anti-inflammatory for migraine: *see* TOLFENAMIC ACID.

Clozaril. Antipsychotic: *see* CLOZAPINE.

Cobadex. Corticosteroid ointment for dermatitis: *see* HYDROCORTISONE, DIMETHICONE.

Cobalin-H. Vitamin B_{12} injection for treatment of B_{12}-deficient anaemia: *see* HYDROXOCOBALAMIN.

Co-Betaloc. Antihypertensive: *see* HYDROCHLOROTHIAZIDE, METOPROLOL.

Codalax. Laxative: *see* CO-DANTHRAMER.

Codafen continus. Combination analgesic with both rapid and sustained release properties: *see* CODEINE, IBUPROFEN.

Codis. Soluble analgesic: *see* CO-CODAPRIN.

Cogentin. Anticholinergic/antiparkinsonian: *see* BENZTROPINE.

Colazide. For ulcerative colitis: *see* BALSALAZIDE

Colestid. For reduction of high blood cholesterol levels: *see* COLESTIPOL.

Colifoam. Corticosteroid in aerosol foam for topical treatment of inflammation of large bowel: *see* HYDROCORTISONE.

Colofac. Antispasmodic for abdominal colic: *see* MEBEVERINE.

Colomycin. Anti-infective: *see* POLYMYXIN B.

Colpermin. Used for intestinal colic: *see* PEPPERMINT OIL.

Coltapaste. Impregnated bandage: *see* COAL TAR, ZINC OXIDE.

Combidol (d). Bile acids for dissolution of cholesterol gall stones: *see* CHENODEOXYCHOLIC ACID, URSODEOXYCHOLIC ACID.

Combivent. For asthma: *see* IPRATROPIUM, SALBUTAMOL.

Combivir. Combination antiviral for use in HIV positive patients with evidence of immunodeficiency: *see* LAMIVUDINE, ZIDOVUDINE.

Comminuted chicken meat (b). For use in carbohydrate and milk protein intolerance in infancy.

Comox. Antibacterial: *see* CO-TRIMOXAZOLE.

Comploment. Sustained-release vitamin preparation for treatment of depression due to pyridoxine deficiency and the oral contraceptive: *see* PYRIDOXINE.

Concavit. Vitamin mixture: *see* ANEURINE, CALCIFEROL, NICOTINAMIDE, PANTOTHENIC ACID, PYRIDOXINE, RIBOFLAVINE, VITAMIN A, VITAMIN C.

Concordin. Antidepressant: *see* PROTRIPTYLINE.

Condyline. Topical treatment for genital warts: *see* PODOPHYLLOTOXIN.

Conotrane. Topical anti-infective: *see* BENZALKONIUM, DIMETHICONE.

Contigen. Treatment for urinary stress incontinence: *see* COLLAGEN.

Convulex. Anticonvulsant: *see* VALPROIC ACID.

Cordarone X. Antidysrhythmic: *see* AMIODARONE.

Cordilox. Antianginal/antihypertensive: *see* VERAPAMIL.

Corgard. Antihypertensive: *see* NADOLOL.

Corgaretic. Antihypertensive: *see* BENDROFLUAZIDE, NADOLOL.

Corlan. Corticosteroid pellet for aphthous ulcers: *see* HYDROCORTISONE.

Coro-nitro. Oral spray for angina pectoris: *see* GLYCERYL TRINITRATE.

Corsodyl. Topical treatment for gingivitis: *see* CHLORHEXIDINE.

Cortisyl. Corticosteroid: *see* CORTISONE.

Corwin. For heart failure: *see* XAMOTEROL.

Cosalgesic. Analgesic: *see* CO-PROXAMOL.

Cosmegen Lyovac. Cytotoxic: *see* ACTINOMYCIN D.

Cosuric. For gout: *see* ALLOPURINOL.

Covering Cream (b). Concealing cream: *see* TITANIUM DIOXIDE.

Covermark (b). Concealing cream: *see* TITANIUM DIOXIDE.

Coversyl. Antihypertensive: *see* PERINDOPRIL.

Cozaar. Antihypertensive: *see* LOSARTAN.

Cozaar-comp. Antihypertensive: *see* HYDROCHLOROTHIAZIDE, LOSARTAN.

Cremalgin. Rubefacient: *see* GLYCOL SALICYLATE, METHYL NICOTINATE, CAPSICUM.

Creon. Used with food in pancreatic insufficiency: *see* PANCREATIC ENZYMES.

Crinone. A vaginal gel to treat infertility and menstrual disorders: *see* PROGESTERONE.

Crixivan. Antiviral for use in HIV positive patients with evidence of immunodeficiency: *see* INDINAVIR.

Cromogen. For asthma: *see* SODIUM CROMOGLYCATE.

Crystapen. Antibiotic: *see* BENZYLPENICILLIN.

Cuplex. Topical treatment for removal of warts, corns and callouses: *see* COPPER ACETATE, SALICYLIC ACID.

Curatoderm. Tropical treatment for psoriasis: *see* TACALCITOL.

Curosurf. Treatment for lung damage (Respiratory Distress Syndrome) in premature babies requiring mechanical ventilation: *see* PORACTANT.

Cutivate. Topical treatment for eczema: *see* FLUTICASONE.

Cyclimorph (c). Narcotic analgesic: *see* CYCLIZINE, MORPHINE.

Cyclogest. Suppository for treatment of premenstrual symptoms: *see* PROGESTERONE.

Cyclo-Progynova. Sex hormones for menopausal symptoms: *see* NORGESTREL, OESTRADIOL.

Cyklokapron. Anti-fibrinolytic: *see* TRANEXAMIC ACID.

Cymevene. Antiviral: *see* GANCICLOVIR.

Cyprostat. Sex hormone for treatment of prostatic carcinoma: *see* CYPROTERONE.

Cystagon. Treatment for rare genetic kidney disorder (cystinosis): *see* CYSTEAMINE.

Cytacon. For vitamin B_{12} deficiency: *see* CYANOCOBALAMIN.

Cytamen. For vitamin B_{12}-deficient anaemias: *see* CYANOCOBALAMIN.

Cytosar. Cytotoxic: *see* CYTARABINE.

Cytotec. For prophylaxis of gastric ulceration caused by non-steroid anti-inflammatory drugs: *see* MISOPROSTOL.

D

Daktacort. Topical anti-infective/corticosteroid: *see* HYDROCORTISONE, MICONAZOLE.

Daktarin. Topical antifungal for skin and nails: *see* MICONAZOLE.

Dalacin C. Antibiotic: *see* CLINDAMYCIN.

Dalivit. Multivitamin preparation: *see* ANEURINE, ASCORBIC ACID, CALCIUM PANTOTHENATE, ERGOCALCIFEROL, NICOTINAMIDE, PYRIDOXINE, RIBOFLAVINE, VITAMIN A, VITAMIN D.

Dalmane. Hypnotic: *see* FLURAZEPAM.

Daneral-SA (d). Anti-allergic: *see* PHENIRAMINE.

Danol. Semisynthetic steroid used in endometriosis: *see* DANAZOL.

Dantrium. Muscle relaxant: *see* DANTROLENE.

Daonil. Oral hypoglycaemic: *see* GLIBENCLAMIDE.

Daraprim. Antimalarial: *see* PYRIMETHAMINE.

Davenol. Decongestant/cough suppressant: *see* CARBINOXAMINE, EPHEDRINE, PHOLCODINE.

DDAVP. Synthetic antidiuretic hormone: *see* DESMOPRESSIN.

Debrisan. Powder used to aid healing of wounds: *see* DEXTRANOMER.

Decadron. Corticosteroid: *see* DEXAMETHASONE.

Deca-Durabolin. Anabolic steroid: *see* NANDROLONE.

De-capeptyl SR. Growth hormone analogue for treatment of advanced prostatic cancer: *see* TRIPTORELIN.

Delfen. Spermicidal contraceptive: *see* NONOXYNOL.

Deltacortril. Corticosteroid tablets or injection: *see* PREDNISOLONE.

Deltacortril Enteric. Corticosteroid. Enteric coating said to reduce gastric irritation: *see* PREDNISOLONE.

Deltastab. Corticosteroid tablets or injection: *see* PREDNISOLONE.

Demser. Antihypertensive: *see* METIROSINE.

Dencyl. Sustained release haematinic: *see* FERROUS SULPHATE, FOLIC ACID, ZINC SULPHATE.

De-Nol. For treatment of peptic ulcer: *see* TRI-POTASSIUM DI-CITRATO BISMUTHATE.

De-Noltab. Antacid, tablet formulation of De-Nol.

Dentomycin. Topical antibiotic for dental use: *see* MINOCYCLINE.

Depixol. Major tranquillizer: *see* FLUPENTHIXOL.

Depo-Medrone. Corticosteroid for intra-articular/intramuscular injection: *see* METHYLPREDNISOLONE.

Deponit 5. Prophylactic antianginal, formulated as a self-adhesive patch for transdermal absorption: *see* GLYCERYL TRINITRATE.

Depo-Provera. Progestogen, depo-injection used in threatened abortion, endometriosis: *see* MEDROXYPROGESTERONE.

Depostat. Progestogen, depo-injection for benign prostatic hypertrophy: *see* GESTRONOL.

Dequacaine. Local anaesthetic lozenges: *see* BENZOCAINE, DEQUALINIUM.

Dequadin. Antiseptic throat lozenges: *see* DEQUALINIUM.

Derbac liquid. Topical anaesthetic cream: *see* CINCHOCAINE.

Dermalex. Soothing antiseptic lotion for prevention of bed sores or urine rash: *see* ALLANTOIN, HEXACHLOROPHANE, SQUALANE.

Dermovate. Topical steroid treatments: *see* CLOBETASOL.

Dermovate-NN. Topical corticosteroid/anti-infective: *see* CLOBETASOL, NEOMYCIN, NYSTATIN.

Deseril. Antiserotoninergic: *see* METHYSERGIDE.

Desferal. Chelating agent: *see* DESFERRIOXAMINE.

Desmospray. Metered nasal spray for treatment of diabetes insipidus and nocturnal enuresis: *see* DESMOPRESSIN.

Desmotabs. For nocturnal enuresis: *see* DESMOPRESSIN.

Destolit. Bile acid for dissolution of cholesterol gall stones: *see* URSODEOXYCHOLIC ACID.

Deteclo. Antibiotic: *see* CHLORTETRACYCLINE, DEMECLOCYCLINE, TETRACYCLINE.

Detrusitol. To control urinary incontinence: *see* TOLTERODINE.

Dettol. Topical antiseptic: *see* CHLOROXYLENOL.

Dexa-Rhinaspray. Nasal spray for allergic or chronic rhinitis: *see* DEXAMETHASONE, NEOMYCIN, TRAMAZOLINE.

Dexedrine (c). CNS stimulant: *see* DEXAMPHETAMINE.

Dextraven 110/150. Plasma expanders: *see* DEXTRANS.

Dextrolyte. Oral electrolyte solution: *see* GLUCOSE, POTASSIUM CHLORIDE, SODIUM LACTATE.

DF 118. Analgesic: *see* DIHYDROCODEINE. (c) injection but not tablets.

DHC Continus. Sustained release analgesic: *see* DIHYDROCODEINE.

Diabinese (d). Oral hypoglycaemic: *see* CHLORPROPAMIDE.

Diamicron. Oral hypoglycaemic: *see* GLICLAZIDE.

Diamox. Diuretic: *see* ACETAZOLAMIDE.

Diamox SR. A sustained release diuretic: *see* ACETAZOLAMIDE.

Dianette. Synthetic sex hormones for use in severe acne in women: *see* CYPROTERONE, ETHINYLOESTRADIOL.

Diarrest. Antidiarrhoeal: *see* CODEINE, DICYCLOMINE, POTASSIUM CHLORIDE, SODIUM CHLORIDE, SODIUM CITRATE.

Diatensec. Diuretic: *see* SPIRONOLACTONE.

Diazemuls. Anxiolytic for injection, formulated as an oil-in-water emulsion. May be used in patients where injection of an aqueous solution causes thrombophlebitis or pain during injection: *see* DIAZEPAM.

Dibenyline. Alpha-adrenoceptor blocker: *see* PHENOXYBENZAMINE.

Diclomax Retard. Sustained-release, non-steroid anti-inflammatory: *see* DICLOFENAC.

Diconal (c). Analgesic: *see* CYCLIZINE, DIPIPANONE.

Dicynene. Haemostatic: *see* ETHAMSYLATE.

Didronel. Used in Paget's disease and osteoporosis: *see* ETIDRONATE DISODIUM.

Differin. Topical treatment for acne: *see* ADAPALENE.

Difflam. Topical, non-steroid anti-inflammatory/analgesic cream: *see* BENZYDAMINE.

Diflucan. Antifungal for oral and vaginal infection: *see* FLUCONAZOLE.

Digibind. Antidote for treatment of life-threatening digoxin toxicity: *see* DIGOXIN-SPECIFIC ANTIBODY.

Dijex. Antacid: *see* ALUMINIUM HYDROXIDE, MAGNESIUM CARBONATE.

Dilzem SR. Sustained-release antihypertensive: *see* DILTIAZEM.

Dimetriose. Synthetic steroid used in endometriosis: *see* GESTRINONE.

Dimotane. Antihistamine: *see* BROMPHENIRAMINE.

Dimotane Co. Cough mixture: *see* BROMPHENIRAMINE, CODEINE, PSEUDOEPHEDRINE.

Dimotane Expectorant. Expectorant cough mixture: *see* BROMPHENIRAMINE, GUAIPHENESIN, PSEUDOEPHEDRINE.

Dimotane Expectorant DC (c). Cough linctus/expectorant. Similar to Dimotane Expectorant plus DIHYDROCODEINE.

Dimotane LA. Sustained-release formulation of Dimotane.

Dimotane Plus. For hayfever and allergic conditions: *see* BROMPHENIRAMINE, PSEUDOEPHEDRINE.

Dimotapp LA. Antihistamine/decongestant for symptomatic treatment of common cold. Available as sustained-release and elixir formulations: *see* BROMPHENIRAMINE, PHENYLEPHRINE, PHENYLPROPANOLAMINE.

Dimyril. Cough suppressant: *see* ISOAMINILE CITRATE.

Dindevan. Anticoagulant: *see* PHENINDIONE.

Dioctyl. Laxative: *see* DOCUSATE SODIUM.

Dioctyl ear drops. Oil for removal of ear wax: *see* DIOCTYL SODIUM SULPHOSUCCINATE.

Dioderm. Corticosteroid cream for inflammatory and allergic skin conditions: *see* HYDROCORTISONE.

Dioralyte. Electrolytes and dextrose supplied in a powder for reconstitution into a solution. Used orally to correct fluid and electrolyte balance (e.g., due to diarrhoea and vomiting).

Diovan. Antihypertensive: *see* VALSARTAN.

Diovol. Antacid: *see* ALUMINIUM. HYDROXIDE, DIMETHICONE, MAGNESIUM HYDROXIDE.

Dipentum. For ulcerative colitis: *see* OLSALAZINE.

Diprobase. Cream or ointment for topical application to dry skin: *see* CETOMACROGOL, CETOSTEARYL ALCOHOL, LIQUID PARAFFIN, SOFT PARAFFIN.

Diprosalic. Ointment and lotion for dermatitis: *see* BETAMETHASONE, SALICYLIC ACID.

Diprosone. Topical corticosteroid: *see* BETAMETHASONE.

Dirythmin-SA. Sustained-release antidysrhythmic: *see* DISOPYRAMIDE.

Disadine. Dry powder spray for skin disinfection: *see* POVIDONE-IODINE.

Disipal. Anticholinergic/antiparkinsonian: *see* ORPHENADRINE.

Disprin CV. Sustained-release analgesic to reduce the risk of thrombosis: *see* ACETYLSALICYLIC ACID.

Distaclor. Antibiotic: *see* CEFACLOR.

Distaclor MR. Sustained-release antibiotic: *see* CEFLACOR.

Distalgesic. Analgesic: *see* DEXTROPROPOXYPHENE, PARACETAMOL.

Distamine. Chelating agent used in rheumatoid arthritis: *see* PENICILLAMINE.

Ditemic. Sustained release haematinic with vitamins: *see* FERROUS SULPHATE, VITAMIN B, VITAMIN C, ZINC SULPHATE.

Dithrocream. Cream for treatment of quiescent psoriasis: *see* DITHRANOL.

Ditropan. Antispasmodic for treatment of urinary complaints: *see* OXYBUTYNIN.

Diumide K. Diuretic with sustained-release potassium: *see* FRUSEMIDE, POTASSIUM CHLORIDE.

Diurexan. Diuretic/antihypertensive: *see* XIPAMIDE.

Dixarit. Migraine prophylactic: *see* CLONIDINE.

Dobutrex. Infusion for treatment of severe heart failure: *see* DOBUTAMINE.

Dolmatil. Antipsychotic: *see* SULPIRIDE.

Dolobid. Analgesic: *see* DIFLUNISAL.

Doloxene. Analgesic: *see* DEXTROPROPOXYPHENE.

Doloxene compound. Analgesic: *see* ACETYLSALICYLIC ACID, CAFFEINE, DEXTROPROPOXYPHENE.

Domical. Antidepressant: *see* AMITRIPTYLINE.

Domperamol. Antiemetic/analgesic for migraine: *see* DOMPERIDONE, PARACETAMOL.

Dopacard. Infusion for treatment of severe heart failure associated with cardiac surgery: *see* DOPEXAMINE.

Dopamet. Antihypertensive: *see* METHYLDOPA.

Dopram. Respiratory stimulant: *see* DOXAPRAM.

Doralese. For relief of the symptoms of prostatic obstruction to urinary outflow: *see* INDORAMIN.

Dostinex. Dopamine agonist used to suppress lactation and other effects of hyperprolactinaemia: *see* CABERGOLINE.

Double Check. Spermicidal contraceptive: *see* NONOXYNOL.

Dovonex. Topical treatment for psoriasis: *see* CALCIPOTRIOL.

Dozic. Tranquillizer: *see* HALOPERIDOL.

Dramamine. Antiemetic: *see* DIMENHYDRINATE.

Drapolene. Topical anti-infective: *see* BENZALKONIUM, CETRIMIDE.

Driclor. Topical antiperspirant for hyperhidrosis: *see* ALUMINIUM CHLORIDE.

Drogenil. Acts against male sex hormone (androgens) in treatment of carcinoma of the prostate gland: *see* FLUTAMIDE.

Droleptan. Premedicant, major tranquillizer: *see* DROPERIDOL.

Dryptal. Diuretic: *see* FRUSEMIDE.

DTIC. Cytotoxic: *see* DACARBAZINE.

Dubam. Rubefacient, pain-relieving spray: *see* ETHYL SALICYLATE, GLYCOL SALICYLATE, METHYL NICOTINATE, METHYL SALICYLATE.

Dulcolax. Laxative: *see* BISACODYL.

Dumicoat. Oral antifungal, in the form of a slow release lacquer applied to dentures: *see* MICONAZOLE.

Duofilm. Topical treatment for warts: *see* LACTIC ACID, SALICYLIC ACID.

Duovent. Bronchodilator for inhalation: *see* FENOTEROL, IPRATROPIUM.

Duphalac. Purgative: *see* LACTULOSE.

Duphaston. For dysmenorrhoea and endometriosis: *see* DYDROGESTERONE.

Duracreme. Spermicidal contraceptive: *see* NONOXYNOL.

Duragel. Spermicidal jelly used for contraception: *see* NONOXYNOL.

Durogesic. Transdermal analgesic patch for treatment of pain in terminal cancer: *see* FENTANYL.

Duromine (c). Anti-obesity: *see* PHENTERMINE.

Dutonin. Antidepressant: *see* NEFAZODONE.

Dyazide. Diuretic combination: *see* HYDROCHLOROTHIAZIDE, TRIAMTERENE.

Dynese. Antacid: *see* MAGALDRATE.

Dyspamet. Gastric histamine receptor blocker; reduces acid secretion: *see* CIMETIDINE.

Dysport. To treat spasms of muscles of the eye and face: *see* BOTULINUM TOXIN A.

Dytac. Diuretic: *see* TRIAMTERENE.

Dytide. Diuretic combination: *see* BENZTHIAZIDE, TRIAMTERENE.

E

E 45 cream. Skin-protective, paraffin-based cream.

Ebufac. Non-steroid anti-inflammatory/analgesic: *see* IBUPROFEN.

Econacort. Topical treatment of fungal/bacterial skin infections: *see* ECONAZOLE, HYDROCORTISONE.

Ecostatin. Antifungal for topical use: *see* ECONAZOLE.

Edecrin. Diuretic: *see* ETHACRYNIC ACID.

Edronax. Antidepressant: *see* REBOXETINE.

Efalith. Topical treatment for seborrhoeic dermatitis: *see* LITHIUM SUCCINATE, ZINC SULPHATE.

Efamast. For treatment of breast pain: *see* GAMOLENIC ACID.

Efcortelan. Topical corticosteroid: *see* HYDROCORTISONE.

Efcortesol inj. Intravenous corticosteroid: *see* HYDROCORTISONE.

Efexor. Antidepressant: *see* VENLAFAXINE.

Effercitrate. Effervescent formulation for treatment of cystitis: *see* POTASSIUM CITRATE.

Effico. 'Tonic': *see* ANEURINE, CAFFEINE, NICOTINAMIDE.

Efudix. Cytotoxic: *see* FLUOROURACIL.

Elantan. Antianginal: *see* ISOSORBIDE MONONITRATE.

Elantan LA. Sustained-release antianginal: *see* ISOSORBIDE MONONITRATE.

Elavil. Antidepressant: *see* AMITRIPTYLINE.

Eldepryl. Used with LEVODOPA in treatment of Parkinson's disease: *see* SELEGILINE.

Eldisine. Cytotoxic: *see* VINDESINE.

Electrolade. Oral replacement for electrolyte and fluid loss due to diarrhoea: *see* GLUCOSE, SODIUM BICARBONATE, SODIUM CHLORIDE, POTASSIUM CHLORIDE.

Electrosol. Soluble tablets for electrolyte depletion: *see* POTASSIUM CHLORIDE, SODIUM BICARBONATE, SODIUM CHLORIDE.

Elemental 028 (b). Dietary substitute for use in malabsorption states and undernourished patients.

Elleste Duet. Hormone replacement therapy for post menopausal symptoms and prophylaxis of post menopausal osteoporosis: *see* OESTRADIOL, NORETHISTERONE.

Ellest Solo. Hormone replacement therapy for post menopausal symptoms and prophylaxis of post menopausal osteoporosis: *see* OESTRADIOL.

Elocon. Topical corticosteroid: *see* MOMETASONE.

Eltroxin. Thyroid hormone: *see* THYROXINE.

Eludril. Antiseptic solution/aerosol for oral infections: *see* AMETHOCAINE, CHLORHEXIDINE, CHLORBUTOL.

Elyzol. Antibiotic dental gel: *see* METRONIDAZOLE.

Emcor. Antihypertensive, antianginal: *see* BISOPROLOL.

Emeside. Anticonvulsant: *see* ETHOSUXIMIDE.

Emflex. Non-steroid anti-inflammatory/analgesic: *see* ACEMETACIN.

Eminase. Intravenous thrombolytic agent for treatment of acute myocardial infarction: *see* ANISTREPLASE.

Emla. Local anaesthetic cream for topical application in children to alleviate the pain of venepuncture: *see* LIGNOCAINE, PRILOCAINE.

Emulsiderm. Soothing, protective skin cream: *see* BENZALKONIUM, LIQUID PARAFFIN.

En-De-Kay. For prevention of dental caries: *see* SODIUM FLUORIDE.

Endoxana. Cytotoxic: *see* CYCLOPHOSPHAMIDE.

Engerix B. Genetically engineered vaccine for immunization against infective hepatitis (Type B): *see* HEPATITIS B VACCINE.

Enrich (b). Liquid feed for enteral absorption.

Ensure. Liquid source of calories for oral nutrition in debilitating conditions.

Entamizole. Amoebicide: *see* DILOXANIDE.

Enteromide. Antibacterial/antidiarrhoeal: *see* CALCIUM SULPHALOXATE.

Entocort CR. Controlled-release oral corticosteroid for treatment of Crohn's disease: *see* BUDESONIDE.

Epanutin. Anticonvulsant: *see* PHENYTOIN.

Ephynal. Tocopheryl: *see* VITAMIN E.

Epilim. Anticonvulsant: *see* SODIUM VALPROATE.

Epivir. Antiviral for use in HIV positive patients with evidence of immunodeficiency: *see* LAMIVUDINE.

Epogam. Fatty acid used in treatment of eczema: *see* GAMOLENIC ACID.

Eppy. Eye drops for glaucoma: *see* ADRENALINE.

Eprex. Hormone treatment for anaemia in chronic renal failure or anaemia caused by chemotherapy: *see* EPOETIN ALFA.

Equagesic. Anti-inflammatory/analgesic: *see* ACETYLSALICYLIC ACID, ETHOHEPTAZINE, MEPROBAMATE.

Equanil (d). Sedative/tranquillizer: *see* MEPROBAMATE.

Erecnos. For intracavernous (penile) injection in treatment of erectile dysfunction: *see* THYMOXAMINE.

Ervevax. Vaccine for immunization against rubella (German measles): *see* RUBELLA VACCINE.

Eryacne. Topical treatment for acne: *see* ERYTHROMYCIN.

Erycen. Antibiotic: *see* ERYTHROMYCIN.

Erymax. Antibiotic: *see* ERYTHROMYCIN.

Erymin. Antibiotic: *see* ERYTHROMYCIN.

Erythrocin. Antibiotic: *see* ERYTHROMYCIN.

Erythroped. Antibiotic: *see* ERYTHROMYCIN.

Eskamel. Cream for acne: *see* RESORCINOL, SULPHUR.

Eskornade. Anticholinergic/sympathomimetic/antihistamine mixture for symptomatic treatment of common cold: *see* DIPHENYLPYRALINE, PHENYLPROPANOLAMINE.

Esmeron. Non-depolarising skeletal muscle relaxant derived from VECURONIUM: *see* ROCURONIUM.

Estracombi. Transdermal patches for HRT: *see* OESTRADIOL, NORETHISTERONE.

Estracyt. Cytotoxic for carcinoma of the prostate: *see* ESTRAMUSTINE PHOSPHATE.

Estraderm. Oestrogen replacement therapy: *see* OESTRADIOL.

Estradurin (d). Sex hormone for carcinoma of the prostate: *see* POLYOESTRADIOL, MEPIVACAINE.

Estrapak. Oestrogen replacement therapy: *see* NORETHISTERONE, OESTRADIOL.

Estring. Hormone for vaginal application in postmenopausal vaginitis: *see* OESTRADIOL.

Ethmozine. Cardiac antiarrhythmic: *see* MORACIZINE.

Ethrane. Inhalational anaesthetic: *see* ENFLURANE.

Ethyol. Cytoprotective used to reduce adverse effects of anticancer drugs: *see* AMIFOSTINE.

Eucardic. Antihypertensive and antianginal: *see* CARVEDILOL.

Eudemine. Antihypertensive/ hyperglycaemic: *see* DIAZOXIDE.

Euglucon. Oral hypoglycaemic: *see* GLIBENCLAMIDE.

Eugynon 30. Oral contraceptive: *see* ETHINYLOESTRADIOL, NORGESTREL.

Eumovate. Corticosteroid eye drops: cream or ointment for skin: *see* CLOBETASONE.

Eumovate-N. As Eumovate plus: *see* NEOMYCIN.

Eumydrin. Anticholinergic: *see* ATROPINE METHONITRATE.

Eurax. Topical antipruritic: *see* CROTAMITON.

Eurax-hydrocortisone. As Eurax plus: *see* HYDROCORTISONE.

Evorel. Transdermal patch for HRT: *see* OESTRADIOL.

Evorel Conti and **Evorel Sequi.** Hormone replacement therapy: *see* OESTRADIOL, NORETHISTERONE.

Exelderm. Topical antifungal for skin infections: *see* SULCONAZOLE.

Exelon. To improve cognitive function in Alzheimer's dementia: *see* RIVASTIGMINE.

Exirel (d). Sympathomimetic bronchodilator: *see* PIRBUTEROL.

Exocin. Topical ophthalmic antibacterial: *see* OFLOXACIN.

Exorex. Topical treatment for psoriasis and other eczematous conditions: *see* COAL TAR.

Exosurf. Treatment for lung damage (Respiratory Distress Syndrome) in premature babies requiring mechanical ventilation: *see* COLFOSCERIL.

Expulin. Cough linctus: *see* CHLORPHENIRAMINE, MENTHOL, PHOLCODINE, PSEUDOEPHEDRINE.

Expurhin. Decongestant linctus: *see* CHLORPHENIRAMINE, EPHEDRINE, MENTHOL.

Exterol. Drops for removal of ear wax: *see* UREA HYDROGEN PEROXIDE.

Eye-Crom. For prophylaxis and treatment of acute and chronic allergic conjunctivitis: *see* SODIUM CROMOGLYCATE.

F

Famvir. Antiviral: *see* FAMCICLOVIR.

Fansidar. Antimalarial: *see* PYRIMETHAMINE, SULFADOXINE.

Fareston. For treatment of breast cancer: *see* TOREMIFENE.

Farlutal. Sex hormone for treatment of hormone-dependent malignancies: *see* MEDROXYPROGESTERONE.

Fasigyn. Antimicrobial: *see* TINIDAZOLE.

Faverin. Antidepressant: *see* FLUVOXAMINE.

Fectrim. Antibacterial: *see* CO-TRIMOXAZOLE.

Fefol Spansule. Slow-release haematinic: *see* FERROUS SULPHATE, FOLIC ACID.

Fefol Z. Sustained-release haematinic: *see* FERROUS SULPHATE, FOLIC ACID, ZINC SULPHATE.

Feldene. Non-steroid anti-inflammatory/analgesic: *see* PIROXICAM.

Femara. For treatment of breast cancer: *see* LETROZOLE.

Fematrix. Transdermal patch for HRT and prevention of osteoporosis: *see* OESTRADIOL.

Femodene. Oral contraceptive: *see* ETHINYLOESTRADIOL, GESTODENE.

Femoseven. Sex hormone for post-menopausal symptoms and prophylaxis of post-menopausal osteoporosis: *see* OESTRADIOL.

Femoston. Sex hormones for post-menopausal symptoms and prophylaxis of post-menopausal osteoporosis: *see* DYDROGESTERONE, OESTRADIOL.

Femulen. Oral contraceptive: *see* ETHYNODIOL.

Fenbid. Sustained-release non-steroid anti-inflammatory/analgesic: *see* IBUPROFEN.

Fenopron. Non-steroid anti-inflammatory/analgesic: *see* FENOPROFEN.

Fentazin. Tranquillizer/antiemetic: *see* PERPHENAZINE.

Feospan Spansule. Slow-release haematinic: *see* FERROUS SULPHATE.

Ferfolic SV. Haematinic: *see* FERROUS GLUCONATE, FOLIC ACID.

Ferrocontin continus (d). Sustained-release haematinic: *see* FERROUS GLYCINE SULPHATE.

Ferrocontin Folic Continus (d). Sustained-release haematinic: *see* FERROUS GLYCINE SULPHATE, FOLIC ACID.

Ferrograd C. Slow-release haematinic/vitamin: *see* FERROUS SULPHATE, VITAMIN C.

Ferrograd Folic. Slow-release haematinic: *see* FERROUS SULPHATE, FOLIC ACID.

Fersaday. Slow-release haematinic: *see* FERROUS FUMARATE.

Fersamal. Haematinic: *see* FERROUS FUMARATE.

Fertiral. Hormone: *see* GONADORELIN.

Fesovit Z. Sustained-release haematinic plus vitamins: *see* ANEURINE, ASCORBIC ACID, FERROUS SULPHATE, NICOTINAMIDE, PYRIDOXINE, RIBOFLAVINE, ZINC SULPHATE.

Flagyl. Antibacterial: *see* METRONIDAZOLE.

Flagyl Compak. Anti-infective: *see* METRONIDAZOLE, NYSTATIN.

Flagyl-S. Antibacterial suspension: *see* BENZOYLMETRONIDAZOLE.

Flamazine. Anti-infective cream for burns: *see* SILVER SULPHADIAZINE.

Flaxedil. Muscle relaxant: *see* GALLAMINE.

Fleet. Enema and oral purgative for use prior to surgery: *see* SODIUM ACID PHOSPHATE.

Fletcher's Enemette. Laxative enema: *see* DOCUSATE SODIUM.

Fletcher's Phosphate Enema. Purgative: *see* SODIUM ACID PHOSPHATE, SODIUM PHOSPHATE.

Flexin continus. Sustained-release non-steroidal anti-inflammatory/analgesic: *see* INDOMETHACIN.

Flixonase. Intranasal steroid for allergic rhinitis: *see* FLUTICASONE.

Flixotide. Corticosteroid inhalation for prevention of asthma: *see* FLUTICASONE.

Flomax MR. For treatment of benign hypertrophy of the prostate gland: *see* TAMSULOSIN.

Florinef. Adrenocorticosteroid: *see* FLUDROCORTISONE.

Floxapen. Antibiotic: *see* FLUCLOXACILLIN.

Fluanxol. Antidepressant/tranquillizer: *see* FLUPENTHIXOL.

Fludara. Cytotoxic: *see* FLUDARABINE.

Fluor-a-Day. For prevention of dental caries: *see* SODIUM FLUORIDE.

Fluorigard. For prevention of dental caries: *see* SODIUM FLUORIDE.

Fluothane. Anaesthetic gas: *see* HALOTHANE.

Fluvirin. Influenza vaccine for immunization.

FML. Corticosteroid eye drops: *see* FLUOROMETHOLONE.

FML-Neo. Topical corticosteroid/antibiotic: *see* FLUOROMETHOLONE, NEOMYCIN.

Folex-350. Haematinic: *see* FERROUS FUMARATE, FOLIC ACID.

Foradil. Selective beta adrenoceptor blocker for treatment of asthma: *see* EFORMOTEROL.

Forceval. Multivitamin and mineral supplement.

Forceval protein (b). Protein, vitamin and mineral supplements for low-sodium/low-fat diets.

Fortagesic. Analgesic: *see* PARACETAMOL, PENTAZOCINE.

Fortral. Analgesic: *see* PENTAZOCINE.

Fortum. Antibiotic: *see* CEFTAZIDIME.

Fortunan. Tranquillizer: *see* HALOPERIDOL.

Fosamax. Biphosphonate to reduce risk of bone fractures in osteoporosis: *see* ALENDRONATE.

Foscavir. Antiviral used to treat cytomegalovirus (CMV) retinitis in patients with AIDS: *see* FOSCARNET.

Fosfor. 'Tonic': *see* PHOSPHORYLCOLAMINE.

Fragmin. Anticoagulant used to prevent blood clotting during haemodialysis or haemofiltration and for treatment of patients with unstable coronary artery disease: *see* HEPARIN.

Franol. Bronchodilator/sedative: *see* EPHEDRINE, THEOPHYLLINE.

Franol expectorant. Bronchodilator/sedative/expectorant. As Franol plus GUAIPHENESIN.

Franol plus. As Franol.

Fre Amine. Amino acids and electrolytes for intravenous nutrition.

Fresubin. Liquid feed. Protein, fat and carbohydrate plus vitamins and electrolytes. For oral feeding when absorption of nutrients and vitamins is impaired.

Frisium. Anxiolytic/anticonvulsant: *see* CLOBAZAM.

Froben. Non-steroid anti-inflammatory analgesic: *see* FLURBIPROFEN.

Fru-Co. Diuretic combination: *see* CO-AMILOFRUSE.

Frumil. Diuretic combination: *see* AMILORIDE, FRUSEMIDE.

Frusene. Diuretic combination: *see* FRUSEMIDE, TRIAMTERENE.

Frusid. Diuretic: *see* FRUSEMIDE.

Fucibet. Topical cream for skin infections: *see* BETAMETHASONE, FUSIDIC ACID.

Fucidin. Antibiotic: *see* FUSIDIC ACID.

Fucidin H oint. and gel. Topical anti-infective/corticosteroid: *see* FUSIDIC ACID, HYDROCORTISONE.

Fucidin Intertulle. Antibiotic gauze dressing: *see* FUSIDIC ACID.

Fulcin 125 and 500. Antifungal: *see* GRISEOFULVIN.

Full Marks. Shampoo for head lice: *see* PHENOTHRIN.

Fungilin. Antifungal: *see* AMPHOTERICIN B.

Fungizone intravenous. Antifungal injection: *see* AMPHOTERICIN B.

Furadantin. Urinary anti-infective: *see* NITROFURANTOIN.

Furamide. Anti-amoebic: *see* DILOXANIDE.

Fybogel. Laxative for diverticular disease, constipation: *see* ISPAGHULA HUSK.

Fybogel mebeverine. Purgative/antispasmodic for treatment of bowel dysfunction and abdominal pain (e.g., irritable bowel syndrome): *see* ISPAGHULA, MEBEVERINE.

Fybozest. To reduce serum cholesterol: *see* ISPAGHULA HUSK.

G

Galactomin Preps (b). Low-lactose dietary supplement.

Galcodine. Cough suppressant: *see* CODEINE.

Galfer and Galfer F.A. For iron and folic acid-deficiency anaemias: *see* FERROUS FUMARATE, FOLIC ACID.

Galfer-Vit. Compound iron and vitamin preparation.

Galpseud. Linctus for hay fever and similar allergic conditions: *see* CHLORPHENIRAMINE, PSEUDOEPHEDRINE.

Gamanil. Antidepressant: *see* LOFEPRAMINE.

Gamimune-N (d). Replacement therapy for congenital gammaglobulin deficiency and for prophylaxis of infection following bone marrow transplantation: *see* IMMUNOGLOBIN G.

Gammabulin. Concentrate of antibodies for prophylaxis against hepatitis A, measles and rubella: *see* IMMUNOGLOBULIN G.

Ganda. Eye drops for glaucoma: *see* GUANETHIDINE.

Garamycin. Antibiotic: *see* GENTAMICIN.

Gardenal sodium (c). Anticonvulsant: *see* PHENOBARBITONE.

Gastrils. Antacid: *see* ALUMINIUM HYDROXIDE, MAGNESIUM CARBONATE.

Gastrobid Continus. Sustained release antiemetic: *see* METOCLOPRAMIDE.

Gastrocote. Antacid: *see* ALGINIC ACID, ALUMINIUM HYDROXIDE, MAGNESIUM TRISILICATE, SODIUM BICARBONATE.

Gastromax. Antiemetic: *see* METOCLOPRAMIDE.

Gastrozepin (d). Selective anticholinergic for treatment of peptic ulcers: *see* PIRENZEPINE.

Gaviscon. Antacid: *see* ALGINIC ACID, ALUMINIUM HYDROXIDE, MAGNESIUM TRISILICATE, SODIUM BICARBONATE.

Gaviscon Liquid. As Gaviscon with CALCIUM CARBONATE.

Gelcosal. Topical treatment for psoriasis or dermatitis: *see* COAL TAR, SALICYLIC ACID.

Gelcotar. Topical treatment for psoriasis: *see* COAL TAR.

Gelofusine. Plasma expander: *see* GELATIN, SODIUM CHLORIDE.

Gelusil. Antacid: *see* ALUMINIUM HYDROXIDE, MAGNESIUM TRISILICATE.

Gemzar. Cytotoxic for treatment of lung cancer: *see* GEMCITABINE.

Genotropin. Synthetic growth hormone for treatment of short stature: *see* SOMATROPIN.

Genticin. Antibiotic for topical and parenteral use: *see* GENTAMICIN.

Genticin HC. As Genticin with HYDROCORTISONE.

Gentisone HC. Anti-inflammatory/anti-infective drops for outer ear: *see* GENTAMICIN, HYDROCORTISONE.

Gentran. Plasma expander: *see* DEXTRANS, SODIUM CHLORIDE.

Gentran 40/Gentran 70. Plasma expanders: *see* DEXTRANS.

Geref. Hormone: *see* SERMORELIN.

Givitol. Compound iron and vitamin preparation.

Glandosane. Solution of cellulose derivative and salts similar to saliva for dry mouth: *see* CARMELLOSE.

Glibenese. Oral hypoglycaemic: *see* GLIPIZIDE.

Glucagen. Hyperglycaemic: *see* GLUCAGON.

Glucobay. Oral hypoglycaemic: *see* ACARBOSE.

Glucophage. Oral hypoglycaemic: *see* METFORMIN.

Glurenorm. Oral antidiabetic: *see* GLIQUIDONE.

Glutarol. Topical treatment for warts: *see* GLUTARALDEHYDE.

Glypressin. Hormone: *see* TERLIPRESSIN.

GoLytely. For rapid bowel clearance prior to examination or surgery: *see* POLYETHYLENE GLYCOL.

Gopten. Antihypertensive: *see* TRANDOLAPRIL.

Graneodin. Antibiotic: *see* GRAMICIDIN, NEOMYCIN.

Granocyte. To raise neutrophil blood cell count in patients undergoing cytotoxic chemotherapy: *see* LENOGRASTIM.

Gregoderm. Topical anti-infective/corticosteroid: *see* HYDROCORTISONE, NEOMYCIN, NYSTATIN, POLYMYXIN B.

Gregovite C. For symptomatic relief of the common cold: *see* CAFFEINE, CODEINE, DIPHENHYDRAMINE, PARACETAMOL, VITAMIN C.

Grisovin. Antifungal: *see* GRISEOFULVIN.

GTN 300. Antianginal/vasodilator: *see* GLYCERYL TRINITRATE.

Guanor. Cough suppressant: *see* AMMONIUM CHLORIDE, DIPHENHYDRAMINE, MENTHOL, SODIUM CITRATE.

Guarem. Dietary aid for treatment of diabetes mellitus: *see* GUAR GUM.

Gyno-Daktarin. Local application for vaginal and penile fungal infections: *see* MICONAZOLE.

Gynol II. Spermicidal jelly used for contraception: *see* NONOXYNOL.

Gyno-Pevaryl. Antifungal for topical treatment of vaginal infections: *see* ECONAZOLE.

H

Haelan. Topical corticosteroid: *see* FLURANDRENOLONE.

Haelan-C. Topical corticosteroid/anti-infective: *see* CLIOQUINOL, FLURANDRENOLONE.

Haemaccel. Plasma expander: *see* GELATIN, SODIUM CHLORIDE.

Halciderm. Topical corticosteroid for skin disorders: *see* HALCINONIDE.

Haldol. Tranquillizer: *see* HALOPERIDOL.

Halfan. Antimalarial: *see* HALOFANTRINE.

Half Securon SR. Sustained-release antihypertensive and antianginal: *see* VERAPAMIL.

Halycitrol. Vitamins for injection: *see* VITAMIN A, VITAMIN D.

Harmogen. Female sex hormones for deficiency states: *see* OESTRONE.

Havrix. Vaccine for immunization against infective hepatitis (Type A): *see* HEPATITIS A VACCINE.

Haymine. For hay fever and similar allergic conditions: *see* CHLORPHENIRAMINE, EPHEDRINE.

Healonid. High-viscosity polymer solution for injection into eye during ophthalmic surgery: *see* SODIUM HYALURONATE.

Hemabate. Synthetic prostaglandin used to treat maternal bleeding after birth: *see* CARBOPROST.

Heminevrin. Sedative/hypnotic: *see* CHLORMETHIAZOLE.

Heparin retard. Anticoagulant formulated for intramuscular or deep subcutaneous injection: *see* HEPARIN.

Hep-flush. Anticoagulant: *see* HEPARIN.

Hepsal. Anticoagulant: *see* HEPARIN.

Herpetad. Antiviral: see ACICLOVIR.

Herpid. Antiviral: *see* IDOXURIDINE, DIMETHYL SULPHOXIDE.

Hespan. Plasma expander: *see* HETASTARCH.

Hexalen. Cytotoxic: *see* ALTRETAMINE.

Hexopal. Peripheral vasodilator: *see* INOSITOL NICOTINATE.

Hibicet hospital concentrate. Antiseptic: *see* CHLORHEXIDINE, CETRIMIDE.

Hibidil. Topical disinfectant to be used undiluted for hand and skin disinfection: *see* CHLORHEXIDINE.

Hibiscrub. Antiseptic cleansing solution for pre-operative preparation of hands: *see* CHLORHEXIDINE.

Hibisol. Topical disinfectant used undiluted for hand and skin disinfection: *see* CHLORHEXIDINE.

Hibitane cream. Antiseptic for prevention of skin infection: *see* CHLORHEXIDINE.

HibTITER. Vaccine: *see* HAEMOPHILUS INFLUENZA TYPE B VACCINE.

Hioxyl. Antiseptic for cleaning infected wounds: *see* HYDROGEN PEROXIDE.

Hiprex. Urinary anti-infective: *see* HEXAMINE.

Hirudoid. Anticoagulant cream for bruising associated with superficial thrombophlebitis or trauma: *see* HEPARIN.

Hismanal. Antihistamine: *see* ASTEMIZOLE.

Histalix. Decongestant: *see* AMMONIUM CHLORIDE, DIPHENHYDRAMINE, MENTHOL, SODIUM CITRATE.

Histryl. Antihistamine: *see* DIPHENYLPYRALINE.

Hivid. Antiviral for use in advanced AIDS: *see* ZALCITABINE.

Honvan. Synthetic sex hormone: *see* STILBOESTROL.

Hormofemin cream. Synthetic sex hormone for pruritis, acne: *see* DIENOESTROL.

Hormonin. Sex hormones for menopausal symptoms: *see* OESTRADIOL, OESTRIOL, OESTRONE.

HRF. For diagnostic use in delayed sexual development and failure of pituitary gland function: *see* GONADORELIN.

Human Insulatard. Semisynthetic human insulin made by biochemical conversion of porcine insulin: *see* INSULIN.

Human Mixtard 30/70. Semisynthetic human insulin made by biochemical conversion of porcine insulin: *see* INSULIN.

Human Monotard. Long-acting synthetic human insulin (zinc suspension): *see* INSULIN.

Human Ultratard. Long-acting human insulin, prepared by modification of porcine insulin: *see* INSULIN.

Human Velosulin. Semisynthetic human insulin made by biochemical conversion of porcine insulin: *see* INSULIN.

Humatrope. Synthetic human growth hormone used to treat growth failure due to growth hormone deficiency: *see* SOMATROPIN.

Humegon (d). For treatment of infertility: *see* HUMAN MENOPAUSAL GONADOTROPHINS.

Humiderm. Emollient cream to treat chronic dry skin conditions: *see* SODIUM PYRROLIDONE-CARBOXYLATE.

Humulin. Human insulins manufactured by genetic engineering using bacteria. Humulin S – soluble insulin, Humulin I – isophane insulin, Humulin Ml/M2 – mixed soluble and isophane insulins, Humulin Zn – insulin zinc suspension: *see* INSULIN.

Hycal. High-calorie (carbohydrate), protein-free liquid for use in protein-free, low-electrolyte diet.

Hycamtin. Cytotoxic for treatment of ovarian cancer: *see* TOPOTECAN.

Hydergine. For impaired mental function in the elderly: *see* DIHYDROERGOTOXINE.

Hydrea. Cytotoxic: *see* HYDROXYUREA.

Hydrenox (d). Diuretic: *see* HYDROFLUMETHIAZIDE.

Hydrocal (d). Topical corticosteroid: *see* CALAMINE, HYDROCORTISONE.

Hydrocortistab. Corticosteroid for parenteral or topical use: *see* HYDROCORTISONE.

Hydrocortisyl. Corticosteroid cream for eczema and other skin conditions: *see* HYDROCORTISONE.

Hydrocortone. Corticosteroid for systemic or topical use: *see* HYDROCORTISONE.

Hydromol. Water-dispersible bath additive for use on dry skin conditions: *see* LIQUID PARAFFIN.

Hydrosaluric. Diuretic: *see* HYDROCHLOROTHIAZIDE.

Hygroton. Diuretic: *see* CHLORTHALIDONE.

Hypercal. Antihypertensive: *see* RAUWOLFIA.

Hypercal B (c). Antihypertensive/ sedative: *see* AMYLOBARBITONE, RAUWOLFIA.

Hypnomidate. Intravenous anaesthetic: *see* ETOMIDATE.

Hypnovel. Intravenous sedative used before and during minor surgery: *see* MIDAZOLAM.

Hypotears. Eye drops for dry eyes: *see* POLYETHYLENE GLYCOL, POLYVINYL ALCOHOL.

Hypovase. Antihypertensive: *see* PRAZOSIN.

Hypurin Bovine. Purified beef insulin: *see* INSULIN.

Hypurin Isophane. Long-acting purified insulin: *see* INSULIN.

Hypurin Lente. Long-acting purified beef insulin (zinc suspension): *see* INSULIN.

Hypurin Neutral. Purified crystalline insulin: *see* INSULIN.

Hypurin Porcine. Purified pork insulin: *see* INSULIN.

Hypurin Protamine Zinc. Long-acting purified insulin: *see* INSULIN.

Hytrin. Antihypertensive: *see* TERAZOSIN.

I J K

Ibugel. Topical non-steroid anti-inflammatory/analgesic: *see* IBUPROFEN.

Ibular. Anti-inflammatory/analgesic: *see* IBUPROFEN.

Ibuspray. Non-steroid analgesic in a metered-dose pump spray: *see* IBUPROFEN.

Icthaband. Topical treatment for eczema: *see* ZINC ICHTHAMMOL.

Iduridin (d). Antiviral: *see* IDOXURIDINE, DIMETHYL SULPHOXIDE.

Ikorel. Anti-anginal: *see* NICORANDIL.

Ilosone. Antibiotic: *see* ERYTHROMYCIN.

Ilube. Eye drops for dry eyes: *see* ACETYLCYSTEINE, HYPROMELLOSE.

Imbrilon. Non-steroid anti-inflammatory/analgesic: *see* INDOMETHACIN.

Imdur. Sustained-release antianginal: *see* ISOSORBIDE MONONITRATE.

Imigran. For acute migraine: *see* SUMATRIPTAN.

Immukin. For treatment of chronic granulomatous disease: *see* INTERFERON GAMMA.

Imodium. Antidiarrhoeal: *see* LOPERAMIDE.

Importal. Laxative: *see* LACTITOL.

Improvera. Sex hormones for post-menopausal symptoms and prophylaxis of post-menopausal osteoporosis: *see* MEDROXYPROGESTERONE, OESTRONE.

Imtack (d). Antianginal available in metered-dose aerosol spray: *see* ISOSORBIDE DINITRATE.

Imunovir. For oral treatment of herpes simplex viral infections: *see* INOSINE PRANOBEX.

Imuran. Cytotoxic: *see* AZATHIOPRINE.

Inderal. Beta-adrenoceptor blocker: *see* PROPRANOLOL.

Inderal LA. Sustained-release antihypertensive: *see* PROPRANOLOL.

Inderetic. Antihypertensive: *see* BENDROFLUAZIDE, PROPRANOLOL.

Inderex. Antihypertensive: *see* BENDROFLUAZIDE, PROPRANOLOL (as in Inderal LA).

Indocid. Non-steroid anti-inflammatory/analgesic: *see* INDOMETHACIN.

Indolar. Non-steroid anti-inflammatory/analgesic: *see* INDOMETHACIN.

Indolar SR. Non-steroid anti-inflammatory/analgesic: *see* INDOMETHACIN.

Indomod. Non-steroid anti-inflammatory/analgesic: *see* INDOMETHACIN.

Infacol. For relief of infantile colic: *see* DIMETHICONE.

Infadrops. Antipyretic for infants: *see* PARACETAMOL.

Influvac. Inactivated influenza virus vaccine.

Innohep. Anticoagulant to treat, or reduce the risk of, thrombosis after surgery: *see* TINZAPARIN.

Innovace. Antihypertensive: *see* ENALAPRIL.

Innozide. Antihypertensive: *see* HYDROCHLOROTHIAZIDE, ENALAPRIL.

Instillagel. Local anaesthetic/antiseptic gel for use in urethral catheterization and cystoscopy: *see* CHLORHEXIDINE, LIGNOCAINE.

Insulatard. Long-acting purified pork (isophane) insulin: *see* INSULIN.

Intal. For asthma: *see* SODIUM CROMOGLYCATE.

Intralgin. Rubefacient/local anaesthetic for muscle pain: *see* BENZOCAINE, SALICYLAMIDE.

Intralipid. High-energy source (fats) for intravenous feeding.

Intraval sodium. Short-acting intravenous barbiturate hypnotic for induction of anaesthesia: *see* THIOPENTONE SODIUM.

Intron A. For treatment of 'hairy cell' leukaemia, non-Hodgkin's lymphoma, malignant melanoma and chronic active hepatitis: *see* INTERFERON ALPHA-2B.

Invirase. Antiviral: *see* SAQUINAVIR.

Iopidine. Alpha$_2$ agonist for control of raised intraocular pressure following laser surgery to the eye: *see* APRACLONIDINE.

Iodosorb. Iodine-releasing preparation used as antiseptic in skin ulcers.

Ionamin (c). Anti-obesity: *see* PHENTERMINE.

Ionil T. Shampoo for dermatitis of scalp: *see* BENZALKONIUM, COAL TAR, SALICYLIC ACID.

Ipral (d). Antimicrobial: *see* TRIMETHOPRIM.

Irofol C. Haematinic for prevention and treatment of anaemia of pregnancy: *see* FERROUS SULPHATE, FOLIC ACID, VITAMIN C.

Isib 60XL. Antianginal: *see* ISOSORBIDE MONONITRATE.

Ismelin. Antihypertensive: *see* GUANETHIDINE.

Ismo 20. Antianginal: *see* ISOSORBIDE MONONITRATE.

Isocard. Antianginal: *see* ISOSORBIDE.

Isogel. Purgative: *see* ISPAGHULA.

Isoket retard. Vasodilator: *see* ISOSORBIDE DINITRATE.

Isomil. Milk-free replacement feed for milk-intolerant patients.

Isopto alkaline. Lubricant ('artificial tears') for dry eyes: *see* HYPROMELLOSE.

Isopto atropine. Long-acting mydriatic eye drops for cycloplegic refraction and uveitis: *see* ATROPINE SULPHATE, METHYLCELLULOSE.

Isopto carbachol. Miotic eye drops for glaucoma: *see* CARBACHOL, HYPROMELLOSE.

Isopto carpine. Miotic eye drops for glaucoma: *see* PILOCARPINE, HYPROMELLOSE.

Isopto frin. Lubricant/decongestant for inflamed (but not infected) eye: *see* METHYLCELLULOSE, PHENYLEPHRINE.

Isopto plain. Lubricant ('artificial tears') for dry eyes: *see* HYPROMELLOSE.

Isordil. Antianginal: *see* ISOSORBIDE DINITRATE.

Isotrex. Topical vitamin A derivative: *see* ISOTRETINOIN.

Isotrexin. Topical treatment for acne: *see* ERYTHROMYCIN, ISOTRETINOIN.

Istin. Antihypertensive/antianginal: *see* AMLODIPINE.

Isuprel. Sympathomimetic injection: *see* ISOPRENALINE.

Jectofer. For iron deficiency anaemia: *see* IRON SORBITOL INJECTION.

Junifen. Antipyretic for febrile conditions in childhood: *see* IBUPROFEN.

Juvela. GLUTEN-free bread/cake mix.

Kabiglobulin. Injection of IMMUNOGLOBULIN G.

Kabikinase. Fibrinolytic: *see* STREPTOKINASE.

Kalspare. Diuretic combination: *see* CHLORTHALIDONE, TRIAMTERENE.

Kalten. Antihypertensive: *see* AMILORIDE, ATENOLOL, HYDROCHLOROTHIAZIDE.

Kamillosan oint. Topical preparation for sore skin: *see* CHAMOMILE OIL.

Kannasyn. Antibiotic: *see* KANAMYCIN.

Kaodene. Antidiarrhoeal: *see* CODEINE, KAOLIN.

Kaopectate. Antidiarrhoeal: *see* KAOLIN.

Karvol. Inhalation for nasal congestion: *see* MENTHOL.

Kay-Cee-L. Potassium supplement: *see* POTASSIUM CHLORIDE.

Kefadim. Antibiotic: *see* CEFTAZIDIME.

Kefadol. Antibiotic: *see* CEPHAMANDOLE.

Keflex. Antibiotic: *see* CEPHALEXIN.

Keftid. Antibiotic: *see* CEFACLOR.

Kefzol. Antibiotic: *see* CEPHAZOLIN.

Kelfizine W. Urinary anti-infective: *see* SULFAMETOPYRAZINE.

Kelocyanor (d). Antidote for cyanide poisoning: *see* DICOBALT EDETATE.

Kemadrin. Antiparkinsonian: *see* PROCYCLIDINE.

Kenalog. Corticosteroid injection for allergic conditions: *see* TRIAMCINOLONE.

Keri. Lotion for dry skin: *see* MINERAL OIL.

Kerlone. Antihypertensive: *see* BETAXOLOL.

Keromask (b). Concealing cream: *see* TITANIUM DIOXIDE.

Kest. Purgative: *see* MAGNESIUM SULPHATE, PHENOLPHTHALEIN.

Ketalar. Anaesthetic: *see* KETAMINE.

Ketovite. Vitamin mixture: *see* ACETOMENAPHTHONE, ANEURINE, BIOTIN, FOLIC ACID, INOSITOL, NICOTINAMIDE,

PANTOTHENIC ACID, PYRIDOXINE, RIBOFLAVINE, VITAMIN C, VITAMIN E.

Ketovite Liquid. As Ketovite with CYANOCOBALAMIN.

Kinidin Durules. Sustained-release antidysrhythmic: *see* QUINIDINE.

Klaricid. Antibiotic: *see* CLARITHROMYCIN.

Klean-Prep. For rapid bowel clearance prior to examination or surgery: *see* POLYETHYLENE GLYCOL.

Kliofem. Female sex hormones for menopausal symptoms (HRT): *see* OESTRADIOL, NORETHISTERONE.

KLN. Antidiarrhoeal: *see* KAOLIN.

Kloref. Effervescent potassium supplement: *see* POTASSIUM CHLORIDE, POTASSIUM BENZOATE, POTASSIUM BICARBONATE.

Kogenate. Recombinant human clotting factor used in treatment of haemophilia: *see* FACTOR VIII.

Kolanticon. Antacid/antispasmodic: *see* ALUMINIUM HYDROXIDE, DICYCLOMINE, DIMETHICONE, MAGNESIUM OXIDE.

Konakion. For prothrombin deficiency: *see* PHYTOMENADIONE.

Konakion MM Paediatric. To prevent haemorrhagic disease in the new born: *see* VITAMIN K.

Konsyl. Laxative: *see* ISPAGHULA.

Kytril. Antiemetic for treatment of nausea and vomiting induced by cytotoxic chemotherapy: *see* GRANISETRON.

L

Labiton. 'Tonic': *see* ANEURINE, CAFFEINE.

Labosept. Oral antiseptic: *see* DEQUALINIUM.

Labrocol. Antihypertensive: *see* LABETALOL.

Lacri-Lube. Lubricant eye ointment for dry eyes: *see* HYDROUS WOOL FAT, LIQUID PARAFFIN.

Lacticare. Skin lotion: *see* LACTIC ACID, SODIUM PYRROLIDONE-CARBOXYLATE.

Ladropen. Antibiotic: *see* FLUCLOXACILLIN.

Lamictal. Anticonvulsant: *see* LAMOTRIGINE.

Lamisil. Antifungal: *see* TERBINAFINE.

Lamprene. Antileprosy: *see* CLOFAZIMINE.

Lanoxin. For cardiac failure: *see* DIGOXIN.

Lanvis. Cytotoxic: *see* THIOGUANINE.

Laractone. Diuretic: *see* SPIRONOLACTONE.

Laraflex. Non-steroid anti-inflammatory/analgesic: *see* NAPROXEN.

Laratrim. Antibiotic: *see* CO-TRIMOXAZOLE.

Largactil. Major tranquillizer/antiemetic/antivertigo: *see* CHLORPROMAZINE.

Lariam. Antimalarial: *see* MEFLOQUINE.

Lasikal. Diuretic with potassium supplement: *see* FRUSEMIDE, POTASSIUM CHLORIDE.

Lasilactone. Combination of two diuretics with different modes of action for use in refractory oedema: *see* FRUSEMIDE, SPIRONOLACTONE.

Lasix. Diuretic: *see* FRUSEMIDE.

Lasix +K (d). Diuretic/potassium supplement: *see* FRUSEMIDE, POTASSIUM CHLORIDE.

Lasma. Sustained-release bronchodilator: *see* THEOPHYLLINE.

Lasonil. Topical treatment for soft tissue injury: *see* HEPARINOID, HYALURONIDASE.

Lasoride. Diuretic combination: *see* AMILORIDE, FRUSEMIDE.

Laxoberal. Purgative: *see* SODIUM PICOSULPHATE.

Ledclair. For heavy metal poisoning: *see* SODIUM CALCIUM EDETATE.

Lederfen. Non-steroid anti-inflammatory/analgesic: *see* FENBUFEN.

Lederfolin. Antagonizes antifolate cytotoxic drugs: *see* FOLINIC ACID.

Ledermycin. Antibiotic: *see* DEMETHYLCHLORTETRACYCLINE.

Lederspan. Corticosteroid injection: *see* TRIAMCINOLONE.

Lenium (b). Shampoo for dandruff: *see* SELENIUM SULPHIDE.

Lentard. Mixture of long-acting purified beef and pork (zinc suspension) insulins: *see* INSULIN.

Lentaron. For treatment of breast cancer: *see* FORMESTANE.

Lentizol. Sustained release. Antidepressant: *see* AMITRIPTYLINE.

Lescol. Used to reduce high blood cholesterol levels: *see* FLUVOSTATIN.

Leucomax. To raise neutrophil blood cell count in patients undergoing cytotoxic chemotherapy and following bone marrow transplantation: *see* MOLGRAMOSTIM.

Leukeran. Cytotoxic: *see* CHLORAMBUCIL.

Leustat. Cytotoxic used to treat leukaemia: *see* CLADRIBINE.

Levophed. Vasoconstrictor: *see* NORADRENALINE.

Lexotan. Anxiolytic: *see* BROMAZEPAM.

Lexpec. Haematinic: *see* FOLIC ACID.

Lexpec with Iron. Haematinic: *see* FERRIC AMMONIUM CITRATE, FOLIC ACID.

Libanil. Oral hypoglycaemic: *see* GLIBENCLAMIDE.

Librium. Anxiolytic: *see* CHLORDIAZEPOXIDE.

Limclair. Increases calcium excretion: *see* SODIUM EDETATE.

Lingraine. Vasoconstrictor for migraine: *see* ERGOTAMINE.

Lioresal. Muscle relaxant: *see* BACLOFEN.

Lipantil. For hyperlipidaemia: *see* FENOFIBRATE.

Lipitor. To reduce blood cholesterol: *see* ATORVASTATIN.

Lipobase. Bland cream for dry skin, eczema and other itchy conditions: *see* CETOMACROGOL, CETOSTEARYL ALCOHOL, LIQUID PARAFFIN, SOFT PARAFFIN.

Lipobay. To reduce serum cholesterol: *see* CERIVASTATIN.

Lipoflavonoid. Multiple vitamins preparation for Ménière's disease.

Lipofundin MCT/LCT and S. Fat emulsion for parenteral nutrition.

Lipostat. To reduce serum cholesterol: *see* PRAVASTATIN.

Lipotriad. Multiple vitamins for retinal degeneration.

Liquifilm tears. Lubricant eye drops for dry eyes: *see* POLYVINYL ALCOHOL.

Liquigen (b). Milk substitute for malabsorption states containing medium-chain triglycerides.

Liskonum. Antidepressant: *see* LITHIUM SALTS.

Litarex. Sustained-release antidepressant: *see* LITHIUM SALTS.

Livial. Steroid with hormonal activity for menopausal disorders: *see* TIBOLONE.

Livostin. Antihistamine nasal spray/eye drops for relief of hayfever symptoms: *see* LEVOCABASTINE.

Locabiotal. Topical antibiotic for infections of upper respiratory tract: *see* FUSAFUNGINE.

Locasol (b). Low-calcium food substitute for calcium intolerance.

Loceryl. Antifungal nail lacquer: *see* AMOROLFINE.

Locoid. Topical corticosteroid for eczema and other skin conditions: *see* HYDROCORTISONE.

Locoid C. Topical corticosteroid/anti-infective: *see* CHLORQUINALDOL, HYDROCORTISONE.

Locoid Crelo. Steroid emulsion for eczema: *see* HYDROCORTISONE.

Locorten-Vioform. Topical corticosteroid/anti-infective for skin or ears: *see* CLIOQUINOL, FLUMETHASONE.

Lodine. Non-steroid anti-inflammatory/analgesic: *see* ETODOLAC.

Loestrin 20. Oral contraceptive: *see* ETHINYLOESTRADIOL, NORETHISTERONE.

Lofenalac (b). Dietary substitute for phenylketonuria.

Logynon. Oral contraceptive: *see* ETHINYLOESTRADIOL, LEVONORGESTREL.

Lomexin. Antifungal for vaginal infection: *see* FENTICONAZOLE.

Lomodex 40 and 70. Plasma expanders: *see* DEXTRANS.

Lomotil. Antidiarrhoeal: *see* ATROPINE SULPHATE, DIPHENOXYLATE.

Loniten. Antihypertensive: *see* MINOXIDIL.

Loperagen. Antidiarrhoeal: *see* LOPERAMIDE.

Lopid. Reduces lipid concentrations in the blood in hyperlipidaemias: *see* GEMFIBROZIL.

Lopresor. Beta-adrenoceptor blocker: *see* METOPROLOL.

Lopresor S.R. Sustained-release formulation of Lopresor: *see* METOPROLOL.

Loron. To treat hypercalcaemia induced by malignant disease: *see* SODIUM CLODRONATE.

Losec. For peptic ulcers and oesophageal reflux: *see* OMEPRAZOLE.

Lotriderm. Cream for topical treatment of cutaneous fungal infections: *see* BETAMETHASONE, CLOTRIMAZOLE.

Loxapac. For acute and chronic psychoses: *see* LOXAPINE.

Lubri-Tears. Lubricating ointment for dry eyes: *see* LIQUID PARAFFIN, SOFT PARAFFIN.

Ludiomil. Antidepressant: *see* MAPROTILINE.

Lustral. Antidepressant: *see* SERTRALINE.

Lyclear. Topical treatment for head lice: *see* PERMETHRIN.

M

Maalox. Antacid: *see* ALUMINIUM HYDROXIDE, MAGNESIUM HYDROXIDE.

Maalox Plus. As Maalox with DIMETHICONE.

Macrobid. Urinary anti-infective: *see* NITROFURANTOIN.

Macrodantin. Antibacterial: *see* NITROFURANTOIN.

Macrodex. Plasma expander: *see* DEXTRANS.

Madopar. Antiparkinsonian: *see* BENSERAZIDE, LEVODOPA.

Magnapen. Antibiotic: *see* AMPICILLIN, FLUCLOXACILLIN.

Malarone. Combination used for treatment of malaria which is resistant to single drug therapy: *see* ATOVAQUONE, PROGUANIL.

Malix. Hypoglycaemic: *see* GLIBENCLAMIDE.

Maloprim. Antimalarials for prophylaxis: *see* DAPSONE, PYRIMETHAMINE.

Manerix. Antidepressant: *see* MOCLOBEMIDE.

Manevac. Laxative: *see* ISPAGHULA, SENNOSIDE B.

Manusept. Topical antiseptic: *see* TRICLOSAN.

Marcain. Local anaesthetic injection: *see* BUPIVACAINE.

Marevan. Oral anticoagulant: *see* WARFARIN.

Marvelon. Oral contraceptive: *see* DESOGESTREL, ETHINYLOESTRADIOL.

Masse (d). Soothing cream for nipples during lactation: *see* ALLANTOIN, AMINOACRIDINE.

Maxamaid (b). Phenylalanine-free mixture of AMINO ACIDS for phenylketonuric patients.

Maxepa. Mixture of fish oils used to reduce plasma lipids in patients with severe hypertriglyceridaemia.

Maxidex. Corticosteroid eye drops for non-infective, inflammatory conditions: *see* DEXAMETHASONE, HYPROMELLOSE.

Maxipro HBV (b). Source of protein for malabsorption states.

Maxitrol. Corticosteroid/antibiotic eye drops/ointment: *see* DEXAMETHASONE, NEOMYCIN, POLYMYXIN B, HYPROMELLOSE.

Maxolon. Antiemetic: *see* METOCLOPRAMIDE.

Maxtrex. Cytotoxic: *see* METHOTREXATE.

MCT (1) and MCT Oil (b). Dietary substitutes containing triglycerides. For use in impaired fat absorption.

Medicoal. Oral adsorbent for treatment of acute poisoning and drug overdose: *see* ACTIVATED CHARCOAL.

Medihaler-Epi. Bronchodilator aerosol: *see* ADRENALINE.

Medihaler-Ergotamine. Aerosol inhalation for migraine: *see* ERGOTAMINE.

Medihaler-Iso/Medihaler Iso-Forte (d). Bronchodilator aerosol: *see* ISOPRENALINE.

Medinex (d). Antihistamine hypnotic: *see* DIPHENHYDRAMINE.

Medised. Analgesic/sedative: *see* PARACETAMOL, PROMETHAZINE.

Medomet. Antihypertensive: *see* METHYLDOPA.

Medrone. Corticosteroid: *see* METHYLPREDNISOLONE.

Mefoxin. Antibiotic: *see* CEFOXITIN.

Megace. Sex hormone: *see* MEGESTROL.

Megaclor (b). Antibiotic: *see* CLOMOCYCLINE.

Melleril. Tranquillizer: *see* THIORIDAZINE.

Mengivac (A + C). Vaccine for immunization against meningitis. Contains inactive groups A and C polysaccharide antigens of Neisseria meningitidis. As Type B meningitis is more common in the U.K., this vaccine is mainly recommended for travel to areas where Types A and C are endemic, e.g. parts of Africa, South America and India.

Menogon. Fertility treatment: *see* MENOTROPHIN.

Menophase. Sex hormones for menopausal disorders: *see* MESTRANOL, NORETHISTERONE.

Menorest. Sex hormone for post-menopausal symptoms: *see* OESTRADIOL.

Meptid. Analgesic: *see* MEPTAZINOL.

Merbentyl. Anticholinergic for gastrointestinal colic: *see* DICYCLOMINE.

Mercilon. Oral contraceptive: *see* DESOGESTREL, ETHINYLOESTRADIOL.

Merieux Tetavax. Purified tetanus toxoid for active immunization against tetanus.

Merocaine. Antiseptic/local anaesthetic lozenge for painful mouth conditions: *see* BENZOCAINE, CETYLPYRIDINIUM.

Merocet. Antiseptic mouthwash or lozenges: *see* CETYLPYRIDINIUM.

Meronem. Antibiotic: *see* MEROPENEM.

Meruvax 11. Live attenuated vaccine for immunization against German measles: *see* RUBELLA VACCINE.

Mestinon. Anticholinesterase: *see* PYRIDOSTIGMINE.

Metabolic Mineral Mixture (b). Dietary mineral supplement.

Metamucil. Purgative: *see* ISPAGHULA.

Metanium. Soothing, protective ointment and powder for nappy rash and other macerated skin conditions: *see* TITANIUM DIOXIDE.

Metatone. 'Tonic': *see* ANEURINE, MANGANESE, POTASSIUM GLYCEROPHOSPHATE, SODIUM GLYCEROPHOSPHATE.

Metazem (d). Antihypertensive: *see* DILTIAZEM.

Metenix 5. Diuretic: *see* METOLAZONE.

Meterfolic. Haematinic: *see* FERROUS FUMARATE, FOLIC ACID.

Metopirone. Used in test of pituitary function: *see* METYRAPONE.

Metosyn. Topical corticosteroid for skin disorders: *see* FLUOCINONIDE.

Metox. Antiemetic: *see* METOCLOPRAMIDE.

Metrodin. Hormone: *see* UROFOLLITROPHIN.

Metrogel. Topical antibiotic treatment for rosacea: *see* METRONIDAZOLE.

Metrolyl. Antimicrobial: *see* METRONIDAZOLE.

Metrotop. Topical gel for reducing smell of fungating tumours: *see* METRONIDAZOLE.

Mexitil. Antidysrhythmic: *see* MEXILETINE.

Mexitil Perlongets. Sustained-release form of Mexitil: *see* MEXILETINE.

Miacalcic. To treat hypercalcaemia associated with Paget's disease or bone cancer: *see* SALCATONIN.

Micolette. Laxative enema: *see* GLYCEROL, SODIUM CITRATE, SODIUM LAURYL SULPHOACETATE.

Micralax. Purgative enema: *see* SODIUM ALKYL SULPHOACETATE, SODIUM CITRATE, SORBIC ACID.

Microgynon 30. Oral contraceptive: *see* ETHINYLOESTRADIOL, NORGESTREL.

Micronor. Oral contraceptive: *see* NORETHISTERONE.

Microval. Oral contraceptive: *see* LEVONORGESTREL.

Mictral. For urinary tract infections: *see* CITRIC ACID, NALIDIXIC ACID, SODIUM BICARBONATE, SODIUM CITRATE.

Midrid. For headache, migraine: *see* DICHLORALPHENAZONE, ISOMETHEPTENE, PARACETAMOL.

Mifegyne. For termination of intra-uterine pregnancy: *see* MIFEPRISTONE.

Migraleve. For migraine: *see* BUCLIZINE, CODEINE, PARACETAMOL.

Migril. Vasoconstrictor for migraine: *see* CAFFEINE, CYCLIZINE, ERGOTAMINE.

Mildison Lipocream. Topical corticosteroid: *see* HYDROCORTISONE.

Minihep. Subcutaneous injection for thromboembolic disease: *see* HEPARIN.

Mini-i-jet. Sympathomimetic: *see* ADRENALINE.

Minims. Single dose ophthalmic preparations.

Minitran. Prophylactic antianginal, formulated as a self-adhesive patch for transdermal absorption: *see* GLYCERYL TRINITRATE.

Minocin. Antibiotic: *see* MINOCYCLINE.

Minodiab. Oral hypoglycaemic: *see* GLIPIZIDE.

Mintec. Enteric coated antispasmodic for relief of pain in irritable bowel syndrome: *see* PEPPERMINT OIL.

Mintezol. Anthelmintic: *see* THIABENDAZOLE.

Minulet. Oral contraceptive: *see* ETHINYLOESTRADIOL, GESTODENE.

Miochol. Solution for intra-ocular irrigation during eye surgery: *see* ACETYLCHOLINE.

Mirena. Intrauterine progestogen-releasing contraceptive system: *see* LEVONORGESTREL.

Mithracin. Cytotoxic: *see* MITHRAMYCIN.

Mitomycin C Kyowa. Cytotoxic: *see* MITOMYCIN.

Mitoxana. Cytotoxic: *see* IFOSFAMIDE.

Mivacron. Muscle relaxant: *see* MIVACURIUM.

Mixtard 30/70. Long-acting purified pork insulin mixture (30 per cent neutral, 70 per cent isophane): *see* INSULIN.

Mizollen. For hay fever and similar allergic conditions: *see* MIZOLASTINE.

M-M-R II. Live vaccine for active immunization against measles, mumps and rubella.

Mobic. Non-steroidal anti-inflammatory for acute osteoarthritis, chronic rheumatoid arthritis and ankylosing spondylitis: *see* MELOXICAM.

Mobiflex. Non-steroid anti-inflammatory/analgesic: *see* TENOXICAM.

Mobilan. Non-steroid anti-inflammatory/analgesic: *see* INDOMETHACIN.

Modalim. Lipid-lowering drug: *see* CIPROFIBRATE.

Modecate. Long-acting tranquillizer injection: *see* FLUPHENAZINE.

Moditen. Tranquillizer: *see* FLUPHENAZINE.

Moditen enanthate. Long-acting tranquillizer injection: *see* FLUPHENAZINE.

Modrasone. Corticosteroid cream and ointment for application to skin: *see* ALCLOMETASONE.

Modrenal. Used to suppress secretion of adrenal cortical hormones: *see* TRILOSTANE.

Moducren. Antihypertensive: *see* AMILORIDE, HYDROCHLOROTHIAZIDE, TIMOLOL.

Moduret 25. Diuretic combination: *see* AMILORIDE, HYDROCHLOROTHIAZIDE.

Moduretic. Diuretic combination. Available as solution for patients who cannot swallow tablets: *see* AMILORIDE, HYDROCHLOROTHIAZIDE.

Mogadon. Hypnotic: *see* NITRAZEPAM.

Molcer. Drops to soften ear wax: *see* DIOCTYL SODIUM SULPHOSUCCINATE.

Molipaxin. Antidepressant: *see* TRAZODONE.

Monclate-P. Clotting factor VIII for treatment of haemophilia. Derived from human plasma which is tested negative for hepatitis B and human immunodeficiency virus.

Monit. Antianginal: *see* ISOSORBIDE MONONITRATE.

Mono-Cedocard. Antianginal: *see* ISOSORBIDE MONONITRATE.

Monocor. Antihypertensive: *see* BISOPROLOL.

Monomax SR. Antianginal: *see* ISOSORBIDE MONONITRATE.

Mononine. Clotting factor concentrate for treatment of Haemophilia B or Christmas Disease: *see* FACTOR IX.

Monoparin. Anticoagulant: *see* HEPARIN.

Monotrim. Antimicrobial: *see* TRIMETHOPRIM.

Monovent. Sympathomimetic bronchodilator: *see* TERBUTALINE.

Monozide 10. Antihypertensive: *see* BISOPROLOL, HYDROCHLOROTHIAZIDE.

Monphytol. Topical antifungal: *see* CHLORBUTOL, METHYL SALICYLATE, SALICYLIC ACID, UNDECENOIC ACID.

Monuril (d). Antibiotic: *see* FOSFOMYCIN.

Morcap SR (c). Sustained release oral narcotic analgesic: *see* MORPHINE.

Morhulin. Topical preparation for abrasions, skin ulcers: *see* ZINC OXIDE.

Motens. Antihypertensive: *see* LACIDIPINE.

Motifene. Rapid release and sustained release non-steroidal, anti-inflammatory analgesic: *see* DICLOFENAC.

Motilium. Antiemetic: *see* DOMPERIDONE.

Motipress. Sedative/antidepressant: *see* FLUPHENAZINE, NORTRIPTYLINE.

Motival. Sedative/antidepressant: *see* FLUPHENAZINE, NORTRIPTYLINE.

Motrin. Non-steroid anti-inflammatory/ analgesic: *see* IBUPROFEN.

Movelat. Rubefacient: *see* CORTICOSTEROID, HEPARINOID, SALICYLIC ACID.

Movicol. Laxative: *see* POLYETHYLENE GLYCOL, POTASSIUM CHLORIDE, SODIUM BICARBONATE, SODIUM CHLORIDE.

MST continus (c). Sustained-release oral narcotic analgesic: *see* MORPHINE.

M.S.U.D. Aid (b). Dietary aid for maple syrup urine disease.

Mucaine. Antacid for oesophageal pain: *see* ALUMINIM HYDROXIDE, MAGNESIUM HYDROXIDE, OXETHAZAINE.

Mucodyne. Mucolytic: *see* CARBOCYSTEINE.

Mucogel. Antacid: *see* ALUMINIUM HYDROXIDE, MAGNESIUM HYDROXIDE.

Multibionta. Intravenous vitamins: *see* ANEURINE, NICOTINAMIDE, PANTOTHENIC ACID, PYRIDOXINE, RIBOFLAVINE, VITAMIN A, VITAMIN C, VITAMIN E.

Multiparin. Anticoagulant: *see* HEPARIN.

Mumpsvax. Live mumps virus vaccine.

MXL (c). Sustained release oral narcotic analgesic: *see* MORPHINE.

Mycardol. Antianginal: *see* PENTAERYTHRITOL TETRANITRATE.

Mycobutin. Antibiotic: *see* RIFABUTIN.

Mycota. Topical antifungal: *see* UNDECENOIC ACID.

Mydriacyl. Mydriatic/cycloplegic eye drops: *see* TROPICAMIDE.

Mydrilate. Mydriatic/cycloplegic eye drops: *see* CYCLOPENTOLATE.

Myleran. Cytotoxic: *see* BUSULPHAN.

Myocrisin. Gold injection for rheumatoid arthritis: *see* AUROTHIOMALATE SODIUM.

Myotonine chloride. Produces gut and bladder emptying: *see* BETHANECHOL.

Mysoline. Anticonvulsant: *see* PRIMIDONE.

N

Nacton/Nacton forte (d). Anticholinergic for peptic ulcers: *see* POLDINE.

Nalcrom. For ulcerative colitis: *see* SODIUM CROMOGLYCATE.

Nalorex. Narcotic antagonist: *see* NALTREXONE.

Napratec. Non-steroid anti-inflammatory/analgesic combined with prophylaxis of gastric ulceration: *see* MISOPROSTOL, NAPROXEN.

Naprosyn. Non-steroid anti-inflammatory/analgesic: *see* NAPROXEN.

Naprosyn SR. Sustained release non-steroid anti-inflammatory/analgesic: *see* NAPROXEN.

Naramig. For migraine: *see* NARATRIPTAN.

Narcan. Narcotic antagonist: *see* NALOXONE.

Nardil. Antidepressant (monoamine oxidase inhibitor): *see* PHENELZINE.

Naropin. Local anaesthetic injection: *see* ROPIVACAINE.

Narphen (c). Analgesic: *see* PHENAZOCINE.

Nasacort. Nasal spray for relief of hay fever symptoms: *see* TRIAMCINOLONE.

Naseptin. Antiseptic/antibacterial cream for topical use in nasal carriers of staphylococci: *see* CHLORHEXIDINE, NEOMYCIN.

Nasobec. Nasal spray for relief of hay fever symptoms: *see* BECLOMETHASONE.

Nasonex. Nasal spray for relief of hayfever symptoms: *see* MOMETASONE.

Natrilix. Antihypertensive: *see* INDAPAMIDE.

Navelbine. For treatment of breast cancer: *see* VINORELBINE.

Navidrex. Diuretic: *see* CYCLOPENTHIAZIDE.

Navispare. Diuretic: *see* AMILORIDE, CYCLOPENTHIAZIDE.

Navoban. Antiemetic: *see* TROPISETRON.

Nebcin. Antibiotic: *see* TOBRAMYCIN.

Negram. Antibacterial: *see* NALIDIXIC ACID.

Neobacrin oint. Topical anti-infective: *see* BACITRACIN, NEOMYCIN.

Neo-cortef. Topical corticosteroid/antibacterial ointment/lotion/drops: *see* HYDROCORTISONE, NEOMYCIN.

Neo-Cytamen. Vitamin: *see* HYDROXOCOBALAMIN.

Neogest. Oral contraceptive: *see* NORGESTREL.

Neo-Mercazole. Antithyroid: *see* CARBIMAZOLE.

Neo-Naclex. Diuretic: *see* BENDROFLUAZIDE.

Neo-Naclex-K. As Neo-Naclex plus POTASSIUM CHLORIDE in slow-release matrix.

Neoral. Immunosuppressant formulated for improved bioavailability: *see* CYCLOSPORIN.

Neorecormon. Hormone treatment for anaemia in chronic renal failure in patients on chronic dialysis: *see* EPOETIN BETA.

Neosporin. Antibacterial eye drops: *see* GRAMICIDIN, NEOMYCIN, POLYMYXIN B.

Neotigason. Used to treat psoriasis: *see* ACITRETIN.

Nephril. Diuretic: *see* POLYTHIAZIDE.

Nericur. Gel for topical treatment of acne: *see* BENZOYL PEROXIDE.

Nerisone. Corticosteroid cream for skin conditions: *see* DIFLUCORTOLONE.

Netillin. Antibiotic: *see* NETILMICIN.

Neulactil. Antipsychotic: *see* PERICYAZINE.

Neupogen. To raise neutrophil blood cell count in patients undergoing cytotoxic chemotherapy: *see* FILGRASTIM.

Neurodyne. Analgesic: *see* CO-CODAMOL.

Neurontin. Anticonvulsant: *see* GABAPENTIN.

Nicorette. Anti-smoking preparations: *see* NICOTINE.

Nicotinell. Transdermal patch for treatment of dependence during withdrawal from cigarette smoking: *see* NICOTINE.

Nidazol. Antimicrobial: *see* METRONIDAZOLE.

Nifelease. Sustained release antianginal, antihypertensive: *see* NIFEDIPINE.

Nifensar XL. Sustained release antihypertensive: *see* NIFEDIPINE.

Niferex. Haematinic: *see* POLYSACCHARIDE-IRON COMPLEX.

Nimbex. Non-depolarising muscle relaxant: *see* CISATRACURIUM.

Nimotop. Intravenous vasodilator used to reduce ischaemia after subarachnoid haemorrhage: *see* NIMODIPINE.

Nipent. Cytotoxic: *see* PENTOSTATIN.

Nitrados. Hypnotic: *see* NITRAZEPAM.

Nitrocine. Antianginal/vasodilator injection. Used as infusion to prevent myocardial ischaemia (e.g., in cardiac surgery or unstable angina): *see* GLYCERYL TRINITRATE.

Nitrocontin. Antianginal: *see* GLYCERYL TRINITRATE.

Nitrolingual. Vasodilator oral spray for symptomatic relief of angina: *see* GLYCERYL TRINITRATE.

Nitromin. Antianginal in spray formulation: *see* GLYCERYL TRINITRATE.

Nitronal. Vasodilator (antianginal) for intravenous use in intractable cardiac failure and unstable angina: *see* GLYCERYL TRINITRATE.

Nivaquine. Antimalarial: *see* CHLOROQUINE.

Nivemycin. Antibiotic for oral and topical use: *see* NEOMYCIN.

Nizoral. Antifungal: *see* KETOCONAZOLE.

NODS. Single dose ophthalmic preparations using a novel ophthalmic delivery system.

Nolvadex. For treatment of anovular infertility and breast cancer: *see* TAMOXIFEN.

Nolvadex-D. As Nolvadex formulated for once-daily dosage: *see* TAMOXIFEN.

Nootropil. Anticonvulsant: *see* PIRACETAM.

Noradran. Bronchodilator expectorant: *see* DIPHENHYDRAMINE, DIPROPHYLLINE, EPHEDRINE, GUAIPHENESIN.

Noratex. Cream for bed sores: *see* COD-LIVER OIL, KAOLIN (light), TALC, ZINC OXIDE.

Norcuron. Muscle relaxant: *see* VECURONIUM.

Norditropin. Synthetic human growth hormone used to treat growth failure due to growth hormone deficiency: *see* SOMATROPIN.

Norgalax. Laxative: *see* DOCUSATE SODIUM.

Norgeston. Oral contraceptive: *see* LEVONORGESTREL.

Noriday. Oral contraceptive: *see* NORETHISTERONE.

Norimin. Oral contraceptive: *see* ETHINYLOESTRADIOL, NORETHISTERONE.

Norinyl-1/Norinyl-1/28. Oral contraceptives: *see* MESTRANOL, NORETHISTERONE.

Noristerat. Depot contraceptive: *see* NORETHISTERONE.

Noritate. Topical treatment for rosacea: *see* METRONIDAZOLE.

Normacol. Purgative: *see* FRANGULA, STERCULIA.

Normasol Undine. Single-dose ophthalmic preparation of SODIUM CHLORIDE.

Normax. Purgative: *see* CO-DANTHRUSATE.

Normegon (d). Hormone injection for use in certain forms of infertility and retarded sexual development: *see* GONADOTROPHIN.

Normetic. Diuretic combination: *see* AMILORIDE, HYDROCHLOROTHIAZIDE.

Normison (d). Hypnotic: *see* TEMAZEPAM.

Norplant. Subdermal long-term depot contraceptive: *see* LEVONORGESTREL.

Norprolac. Dopamine antagonist used in suppression of the effects of hyperprolactinaemia, e.g. galactorrhoea: *see* QUINAGOLIDE.

Novantrone. Cytotoxic: *see* MITOZANTRONE.

Norvir. Antiviral: *see* RITONAVIR.

Novoseven. Recombinant Coagulation Factor used to stop bleeding in patients with haemophilia (deficiency of clotting factor VIII): *see* COAGULATION FACTOR VIIA.

Noxyflex S. Anti-infective for instillation in bladder or other body cavities: *see* NOXYTHIOLINE.

Noxyflex with amethocaine. As Noxyflex S plus AMETHOCAINE as local anaesthetic.

Nozinan. Antipsychotic: *see* METHOTRIMEPRAZINE.

Nubain. Analgesic: *see* NALBUPHINE.

Nuelin. Bronchodilator: *see* THEOPHYLLINE.

Nulacin. Antacid: *see* CALCIUM AND MAGNESIUM ANTACIDS.

Nupercainal. Topical skin anaesthetic: *see* CINCHOCAINE.

Nurofen. Non-prescription analgesic: *see* IBUPROFEN.

Nu-Seals Aspirin. Enteric-coated analgesic: *see* ACETYLSALICYLIC ACID.

Nutramigen (b). Dietary aid for lactose intolerance, galactosaemia.

Nutraplus. Topical cream for dry skin: *see* UREA.

Nutrizym. For use in pancreatic deficiency: *see* PANCREATIC ENZYMES.

Nuvelle. Hormone replacement therapy: *see* LEVONORGESTREL, OESTRADIOL.

Nycopren. Non-steroid anti-inflammatory/analgesic: *see* NAPROXEN.

Nyspes. Antifungal pessaries: *see* NYSTATIN.

Nystadermal. Topical antifungal/anti-inflammatory: *see* NYSTATIN, TRIAMCINOLONE.

Nystaform. Cream or ointment for topical treatment of fungal skin infections due to *Candida* spp.: *see* CHLORHEXIDINE, NYSTATIN.

Nystaform-HC. Topical anti-infective/anti-inflammatory: *see* CHLORHEXIDINE, HYDROCORTISONE, NYSTATIN.

Nystan. Antifungal: *see* NYSTATIN.

Nytol. A hypnotic: *see* DIPHENHYDRAMINE.

O

Occlusal. Wart remover: *see* SALICYLIC ACID.

Octovit. Multi-vitamin and mineral supplement: *see* ASCORBIC ACID, CHOLECALCIFEROL, CYANOCOBALAMIN, NICOTINAMIDE, PYRIDOXINE, RIBOFLAVINE, THIAMINE, VITAMIN A, VITAMIN E; plus CALCIUM HYDROGEN PHOSPHATE, FERROUS SULPHATE, MAGNESIUM HYDROXIDE, ZINC SULPHATE.

Ocufen. Eye drops to prevent trauma-induced pupil constriction during eye surgery: *see* FLURBIPROFEN.

Ocusert Pilo. Topical sustained-release treatment for glaucoma. The drug is contained within a membrane in single dose units which are placed under the eyelid: *see* PILOCARPINE.

Odrik. Antihypertensive: *see* TRANDOLAPRIL.

Oestrogel. Sex hormone for post-menopausal symptoms: *see* OESTRADIOL.

Olbetam. Reduces raised blood lipids: *see* ACIPIMOX.

Omnopon-Scopolamine (c). Narcotic analgesic/anticholinergic for use prior to operation: *see* HYOSCINE HYDROBROMIDE, PAPAVERETUM.

Oncovin. Cytotoxic: *see* VINCRISTINE.

One-Alpha. Hormone: *see* ALPHA-CALCIDOL.

Operidine (c) (d). Narcotic analgesic: *see* PHENOPERIDINE.

Ophthaine. Topical ophthalmic anaesthetic: *see* PROXYMETACAINE.

Opilon. Peripheral vasodilator: *see* THYMOXAMINE.

Opticrom. Eye drops for allergic conjunctivitis: *see* SODIUM CROMOGLYCATE.

Optilast. Antihistamine eye drops for allergic conjunctivitis: *see* AZELASTINE.

Optimax. Antidepressant: *see* TRYPTOPHAN.

Optimine. Antihistamine: *see* AZATADINE.

Orabase. Topical inert protective application for skin and mucosae.

Orabet. Oral hypoglycaemic: *see* METFORMIN.

Orahesive. Topical inert protective powder for skin and mucosae.

Oraldene. Rinse for oral infections: *see* HEXETIDINE.

Oramorph. Liquid, oral analgesic: *see* MORPHINE.

Orap. Tranquillizer: *see* PIMOZIDE.

Orbenin. Antibiotic: *see* CLOXACILLIN.

Orelox. Antibiotic: *see* CEFPODOXIME.

Orgafol (d). For treatment of infertility: *see* UROFOLLITROPHIN.

Orgaran. Anticoagulant: *see* DANAPAROID SODIUM.

Orimeten. Cytotoxic: *see* AMINOGLUTETHIMIDE.

Orovite. Vitamin mixture: *see* ANEURINE, NICOTINAMIDE, PYRIDOXINE, RIBOFLAVINE, VITAMIN C.

Orovite 7. Vitamin mixture for deficiency: *see* ANEURINE, CALCIFEROL, NICOTINAMIDE, PYRIDOXINE, RIBOFLAVINE, VITAMIN A, VITAMIN C.

Ortho-Creme. Spermicidal cream: *see* NONOXYNOL, RICINOLEIC ACID, SODIUM LAURYL SULPHATE.

Ortho-Forms. Spermicidal pessary.

Ortho-Gynest. Vaginal pessary for vaginal inflammation and irritation: *see* OESTRIOL.

Ortho-Novin. Oral contraceptive: *see* MESTRANOL, NORETHISTERONE.

Orudis. Non-steroid anti-inflammatory/analgesic: *see* KETOPROFEN.

Oruvail. Sustained-release non-steroid anti-inflammatory/analgesic: *see* KETOPROFEN.

Osmolite (b). Liquid feed for enteral absorption.

Ossopan. Source of calcium and fluoride for bone and dental states.

Ostersoy. Substitute for cow's milk in infant feeds. For use in intolerance to cow's milk, sucrose and lactose. Contains carbohydrate (from corn syrup), fat (from vegetable oils), and protein (from soya), together with vitamins and minerals.

Ostram. For osteoporosis and calcium deficiency: *see* CALCIUM PHOSPHATE.

Otomize. Spray for treatment of external ear inflammation/infection: *see* DEXAMETHASONE, NEOMYCIN.

Otosporin. Antibiotic/anti-inflammatory ear drops: *see* HYDROCORTISONE, NEOMYCIN, POLYMYXIN B.

Otrivine. Nasal decongestant: *see* XYLOMETAZOLINE.

Ovestin. Female sex hormone for deficiency states: *see* OESTRIOL.

Ovran. Oral contraceptive: *see* ETHINYLOESTRADIOL, NORGESTREL.

Ovranette. Oral contraceptive: *see* ETHINYLOESTRADIOL, NORGESTREL.

Ovysmen. Oral contraceptive: *see* ETHINYLOESTRADIOL, NORETHISTERONE.

Oxanid. Anxiolytic: *see* OXAZEPAM.

Oxivent. Bronchodilator: *see* OXITROPIUM.

Oxymycin. Antibiotic: *see* OXYTETRACYCLINE.

P

Pabrinex. Vitamin injection: *see* VITAMIN B, VITAMIN C.

Paediasure (b). Oral dietary supplement for children up to six years old.

Paldesic. Analgesic elixir: *see* PARACETAMOL.

Palfium (c). Narcotic analgesic: *see* DEXTROMORAMIDE.

Palladone. Opioid analgesic for severe pain: *see* HYDROMORPHONE.

Paludrine. Antimalarial: *see* PROGUANIL.

Pamergan P100 (c). Premedication combination containing narcotic analgesic: *see* PETHIDINE, PROMETHAZINE.

Pameton. Analgesic with antidote against overdose: *see* METHIONINE, PARACETAMOL.

Panadeine. Non-prescription analgesic: *see* CODEINE, PARACETAMOL.

Panadol. Analgesic: *see* CODEINE, PARACETAMOL.

Pancrease. *See* PANCREATIC ENZYMES.

Pancrex/Pancrex V/Pancrex V Forte. For use in pancreatic deficiency: *see* PANCREATIN.

Panoxyl 5 and 10. Topical treatment for acne: *see* BENZOYL PEROXIDE.

Papulex. Anti-inflammatory for topical treatment of acne: *see* NICOTINAMIDE.

Paracodol. Effervescent analgesic/antipyretic: *see* CODEINE, PARACETAMOL.

Parake. Analgesic/antipyretic: *see* CO-CODAMOL.

Paramax. Analgesic/antiemetic for migraine. METOCLOPRAMIDE aids drug absorption by relief of the gastric stasis which can occur during a migraine attack as well as acting as an antiemetic: *see* METOCLOPRAMIDE, PARACETAMOL.

Paramol. Analgesic: *see* DIHYDROCODEINE, PARACETAMOL.

Paraplatin. Cytotoxic: *see* CARBOPLATIN.

Parlodel. Dopamine agonist: *see* BROMOCRIPTINE.

Parmid. Antiemetic: *see* METOCLOPRAMIDE.

Parnate. Antidepressant monoamine oxidase inhibitor: *see* TRANYLCYPROMINE.

Paroven. Vitamin derivative for symptomatic treatment of aching associated with varicose veins: *see* TROXERUTIN.

Parstelin. Antidepressant monoamine oxidase inhibitor/tranquillizer: *see* TRANYLCYPROMINE, TRIFLUOPERAZINE.

Partobulin. To prevent sensitization from rhesus (D) incompatibility: *see* ANTI-D IMMUNOGLOBULIN.

Parvolex. Injection for treatment of paracetamol overdosage: *see* ACETYLCYSTEINE.

Pavacol-D. Cough suppressant: *see* ESSENTIAL OILS, PHOLCODINE.

Pavulon. Muscle relaxant: *see* PANCURONIUM.

Paxadon. Vitamin: *see* PYRIDOXINE.

Paxalgesic. Analgesic: *see* CO-PROXAMOL.

Paxane. Hypnotic: *see* FLURAZEPAM.

Paxofen. Non-steroid anti-inflammatory/analgesic: *see* IBUPROFEN.

Pecram. Sustained release bronchodilator: *see* AMINOPHYLLINE.

Ped-El. Electrolytes and trace elements for parenteral nutrition.

Penbritin. Antibiotic: *see* AMPICILLIN.

Pendramine. Chelating agent: *see* PENICILLAMINE.

Pentacarinat. Antiprotozoal: *see* PENTAMIDINE.

Pentasa. Enema to treat ulcerative colitis: *see* MESALAZINE.

Pentostam. Antimony derivative: *see* STIBOGLUCONATE SODIUM.

Pepcid PM. Gastric histamine blocker; reduces acid secretions: *see* FAMOTIDINE.

Peptamen (b). Peptide based liquid food for use when gastrointestinal function is impaired. Contains carbohydrate (maltodextrin and starch), protein (whey protein hydrolysate), fat (MCT, sunflower oil, lecithin and residual milk fat), vitamins, minerals and trace elements.

Pepti-2000 LF. Dietary aid. Predigested carbohydrates, proteins, fats and vitamins for oral feeding when there is malabsorption.

Percutol. Vasodilator gel for application to skin in prophylaxis of angina: *see* GLYCERYL TRINITRATE.

Perdix. Antihypertensive: *see* MOEXIPRIL.

Perfan. For relief of cardiac failure: *see* ENOXIMONE.

Pergonal. Hormone: *see* MENOTROPHIN.

Periactin. Serotonin antagonist for stimulation of appetite: *see* CYPROHEPTADINE.

Perinal. For itching and pain from haemorrhoids: *see* HYDROCORTISONE, LIGNOCAINE.

Persantin. For ischaemic heart disease: *see* DIPYRIDAMOLE.

Pevaryl. Topical antifungal for skin infections: *see* ECONAZOLE, TRIAMCINOLONE.

Pharmalgen. Insect venom, prepared from bees or wasps for desensitization in allergic individuals.

Pharmorubicin. Cytotoxic: *see* EPIRUBICIN.

Phasal. Sustained-release antimanic: *see* LITHIUM SALTS.

Phenergan. Antihistamine for topical and systemic use: *see* PROMETHAZINE.

Phiso-Med. Anti-infective for cleansing skin/hair: *see* CHLORHEXIDINE.

Phosphate-Sandoz. Effervescent phosphate supplement for hyperparathyroidism and other bone disease.

Phyllocontin. For asthma and cardiac failure: *see* AMINOPHYLLINE.

Physeptone (c). Narcotic analgesic: *see* METHADONE.

Physiotens. Antihypertensive: *see* MOXONIDINE.

Phytex. Topical antifungal paint: *see* BORIC ACID, METHYL SALICYLATE, SALICYLIC ACID, TANNIC ACID.

Phytocil Powder. Topical antifungal: *see* CHLOROPHENOXYETHANOL, MENTHOL, PHENOXYPROPANOL, ZINC UNDECENOATE.

Picolax. Saline purgative: *see* MAGNESIUM CITRATE, SODIUM PICOSULPHATE.

Pilogel. Miotic eye gel for glaucoma: *see* PILOCARPINE.

Piportil depot. Long-acting tranquillizer injection: *see* PIPOTHIAZINE.

Pipril. Parenteral antibacterial: *see* PIPERACILLIN.

Piriton. Antihistamine: *see* CHLORPHENIRAMINE.

Pitressin. Hormone: *see* VASOPRESSIN.

P.K. Aid 1 (b). Dietary aid for phenylketonuria.

Plaquenil. Anti-inflammatory: *see* HYDROXYCHLOROQUINE.

Plendil. Antianginal/antihypertensive: *see* FELODIPINE.

Plesmet. For iron-deficiency anaemia: *see* FERROUS SULPHATE.

Pneumovax II. Vaccine for immunization against pneumococcal infections e.g. lobar pneumonia, meningitis or endocarditis.

Polycal (b). Source of carbohydrate for kidney, liver, and various metabolic diseases.

Polycose (b). Lactose- and GLUTEN-free polysaccharide mixture.

Polyfax. Antibiotic: *see* BACITRACIN, POLYMYXIN B.

Polytar (b). Topical treatment for psoriasis: *see* COAL TAR.

Polytrim. Antibacterial eye drops: *see* POLYMYXIN B, TRIMETHOPRIM.

Ponderax (d). Anti-obesity: *see* FENFLURAMINE.

Pondocillin. Antibiotic: *see* PIVAMPICILLIN.

Ponstan. Anti-inflammatory/analgesic: *see* MEFENAMIC ACID.

Posalfilin. Topical treatment for warts: *see* PODOPHYLLUM, SALICYLIC ACID.

Posiject. Infusion for treatment of severe heart failure: *see* DOBUTAMINE.

Posicor. Antihypertensive: *see* MIBEFRADIL.

postMI. Enteric-coated aspirin to reduce the risk of thrombosis: *see* ACETYLSALICYLIC ACID.

Potaba. Non-steroid anti-inflammatory: *see* POTASSIUM *para*-AMINOBENZOATE.

Powergel. Topical anti-inflammatory analgesic: *see* KETOPROFEN.

Pragmatar. Topical treatment for seborrhoea: *see* COAL TAR, SALICYLIC ACID, SULPHUR.

Praxilene. Peripheral vasodilator: *see* NAFTIDROFURYL.

Precortisyl. Corticosteroid: *see* PREDNISOLONE.

Predenema. Corticosteroid enema: *see* PREDNISOLONE.

Predfoam. Corticosteroid aerosol foam for rectal administration. Used to treat ulcerative colitis and similar inflammatory bowel conditions: *see* PREDNISOLONE.

Pred Forte. Topical corticosteroid eye drops for use in inflammatory non-infective eye conditions: *see* PREDNISOLONE.

Prednesol. Corticosteroid: *see* PREDNISOLONE.

Predsol. Corticosteroid: *see* PREDNISOLONE.

Predsol-N. Corticosteroid/antibiotic ear drops: *see* NEOMYCIN, PREDNISOLONE.

Pregaday. For anaemia of pregnancy: *see* FERROUS FUMARATE, FOLIC ACID.

Pregestimil (b). Dietary aid for glucose, lactose, protein intolerance.

Premarin. Natural oestrogens from pregnant mare's urine for deficiency states.

Premique. Sex hormones for post-menopausal symptoms: *see* MEDROXYPROGESTERONE, OESTROGEN.

Prempak-C. Sex hormones for replacement therapy at and after menopause: *see* NORGESTREL, OESTROGEN.

Prepulsid. For treatment of gastric reflux and delayed gastric emptying: *see* CISAPRIDE.

Prescal. Antihypertensive: *see* ISRADIPINE.

Preservex. Non-steroidal anti-inflammatory analgesic: *see* ACECLOFENAC.

Pressimmune. Anti-human lymphocyte globulin for immunosuppression.

Prestim. Antihypertensive: *see* BENDROFLUAZIDE, TIMOLOL.

Priadel. Antidepressant: *see* LITHIUM SALTS.

Primacor. Phosphodiesterase inhibitor for treatment of severe congestive cardiac failure: *see* MILRINONE.

Primalan. Antihistamine: *see* MEQUITAZINE.

Primaxin. Antibiotic for intravenous use: *see* CILASTIN, IMIPENEM.

Primolut N. To reduce or postpone menstruation: *see* NORETHISTERONE.

Primoteston depot. Male sex hormone for deficiency states: *see* TESTOSTERONE.

Primperan. Antiemetic. Promotes gastric emptying: *see* METOCLOPRAMIDE.

Prioderm. Topical treatment for lice: *see* MALATHION.

Pripsen. For threadworms, roundworms: *see* PIPERAZINE.

Pro-Banthine. Anticholinergic used for antispasmodic and antacid effects: *see* PROPANTHELINE.

Proctofoam HC. Topical treatment for ano-rectal conditions: *see* HYDROCORTISONE, PRAMOXINE.

Proctosedyl. Local treatment for haemorrhoids: *see* CINCHOCAINE, HYDROCORTISONE.

Profasi. Hormone injection for use in certain forms of infertility and retarded sexual development: *see* CHORIONIC GONADOTROPHIN.

Proflex. Non-steroidal anti-inflammatory analgesic for topical use: *see* IBUPROFEN.

Progynova. Female sex hormone for deficiency states: *see* OESTRADIOL.

Proleukin. Cytotoxic: *see* ALDESLEUKIN.

Proluton Depot. Hormone injection for prevention of habitual abortion: *see* HYDROXYPROGESTERONE.

Prominal. Anticonvulsant: *see* METHYLPHENOBARBITONE.

Pronestyl. Antidysrhythmic: *see* PROCAINAMIDE.

Pronoxen Continus. Sustained release non-steroid anti-inflammatory/analgesic: *see* NAPROXEN.

Propaderm. Topical corticosteroid: *see* BECLOMETHASONE.

Propaderm A and C. Topical corticosteroid/anti-infective: *see* BECLOMETHASONE, CHLORTETRACYCLINE, CLIOQUINOL.

Propain. Analgesic/antihistamine for headache and muscular pain: *see* CAFFEINE, CODEINE, DIPHENHYDRAMINE, PARACETAMOL.

Propanix LA. Antihypertensive: *see* PROPRANOLOL

Propine. Eye drops for chronic open-angle glaucoma: *see* DIPIVEFRINE.

Proscar. For treatment of benign hypertrophy of the prostate gland: *see* FINASTERIDE.

Prosobee (b). Dietary aid for lactose intolerance.

Prostap SR. Hormone used to treat cancer of the prostate and before surgery of the uterus: *see* LEUPRORELIN.

Prostin E2. Prostaglandin: *see* DINOPROSTONE.

Prostin F2 Alpha. Prostaglandin: *see* DINOPROST.

Prostin VR. Prostaglandin: *see* ALPROSTADIL.

Prothiaden. Antidepressant: *see* DOTHIEPIN.

Protifar. Dietary aid. High-protein source from skimmed milk for use in low-protein states.

Protium. For peptic ulcers and oesophageal reflux: *see* PANTOPRAZOLE.

Provera. For menstrual disorders and prevention of threatened abortion: *see* MEDROXYPROGESTERONE.

Provera 100 mg. High-dose MEDROXYPROGESTERONE for treatment of endometrial carcinoma or hypernephroma.

Provigil. To reduce sedation in narcolepsy: *see* MODAFINIL.

Pro-Viron. Male sex hormone for deficiency states: *see* MESTEROLONE.

Prozac. Antidepressant: *see* FLUOXETINE.

P.R. Spray. Antidepressant: *see* CHLOROFLUOROMETHANE.

Psoriderm preps. Topical treatments for psoriasis: *see* COAL TAR, LECITHINS.

Psoriderm-S. As Psoriderm plus SALICYLIC ACID.

Psorigel. Topical solution for psoriasis: *see* COAL TAR.

Psorin. For topical treatment of psoriasis and eczema: *see* COAL TAR, DITHRANOL, SALICYLIC ACID.

Pulmadil (d). Bronchodilator aerosol: *see* RIMITEROL.

Pulmicort. Steroid aerosol for asthma: *see* BUDESONIDE.

Pulmozyme. Synthetic enzyme used to reduce sputum viscosity in cases of cystic fibrosis: *see* DORNASE ALFA.

Pump-Hep. Anticoagulant for continuous infuson: *see* HEPARIN.

Puri-Nethol. Cytotoxic: *see* MERCAPTOPURINE.

Pylorid. For treatment of peptic ulcers where there is evidence of bacterial infection due to *Helicobacter pylori*: *see* RANITIDINE BISMUTH CITRATE.

Pyralvex. Topical anti-inflammatory for mouth ulcers: *see* ANTHRAQUINONE, GLYCOSIDES, SALICYLIC ACID.

Pyrogastrone. For oesophagitis due to gastric reflux: *see* ALUMINIUM HYDROXIDE, CARBENOXOLONE, MAGNESIUM TRISILICATE, SODIUM BICARBONATE.

Q R

Quellada M. Topical treatment for scabies and lice: *see* MALATHION.

Questran. For hypercholesterolaemia: *see* CHOLESTYRAMINE.

Quinaband. Impregnated bandage: *see* CALAMINE, CLIOQUINOL, ZINC OXIDE.

Quinocort. Anti-infective/corticosteroid cream for topical treatment of infected eczema and similar skin conditions: *see* HYDROCORTISONE, HYDROXYQUINOLINE.

Quinoderm. Topical treatment for acne: *see* BENZOYL PEROXIDE, HYDROXYQUINOLINE.

Quinoped. Topical antifungal for feet: *see* BENZOYL PEROXIDE, HYDROXYQUINOLINE.

Radian B. Rubefacient: *see* ACETYLSALICYLIC ACID, METHYL SALICYLATE, MENTHOL, CAMPHOR.

Rapifen (d). Narcotic analgesic: *see* ALFENTANIL.

Rapitard (d). Long-acting mixture of purified beef and pork insulins: *see* INSULIN.

Rapitil. Eye drops for allergic conjunctivitis: *see* NEDOCROMIL.

Rastinon. Hypoglycaemic: *see* TOLBUTAMIDE.

Raxar. Antibiotic: *see* GREPAFLOXACIN.

RBC. Topical antihistamine: *see* ANTAZOLINE, CALAMINE, CAMPHOR, CETRIMIDE.

Rebif. For reduction of frequency and severity of relapses in multiple sclerosis: *see* INTERFERON BETA-1A.

Recombinate. Clotting factor for treatment of haemophilia: *see* FACTOR VIII.

Refludan. Anticoagulant: *see* LEPIRUDIN.

Refolinon. Antagonizes antifolate cytotoxic drugs: *see* FOLINIC ACID.

Regaine. Topical treatment for male-pattern baldness: *see* MINOXIDIL.

Regulan. Purgative: *see* ISPAGHULA.

Rehidrat. Electrolytes and sugars supplied in a powder for reconstitution into solution. Used orally to correct fluid and electrolyte imbalance (e.g., due to diarrhoea and vomiting).

Relaxit. Enema for constipation: *see* GLYCEROL, SODIUM CITRATE, SODIUM LAURYL SULPHATE, SORBIC ACID, SORBITOL.

Relefact LH-RH. For diagnostic use in delayed sexual development and failure of pituitary gland function: *see* GONADORELIN.

Relifex. Non-steroid anti-inflammatory analgesic: *see* NABUMETONE.

Remedeine. Analgesic: *see* DIHYDROCODEINE, PARACETAMOL.

Remnos. Hypnotic: *see* NITRAZEPAM.

Reopro. Monoclonal antibody used to reduce risk of blood clotting after heart surgery and as an antianginal: *see* ABCIXIMAB.

Requip. Dopamine agonist for treatment of Parkinson's Disease: *see* ROPINIROLE.

Resonium-A. Ion exchange resin: *see* SODIUM POLYSTYRENE SULPHONATE.

Respacal. Bronchodilator: *see* TULOBUTEROL.

Respontin Nebules. Bronchodilator nebuliser: *see* IPATROPIUM.

Restandol. Male sex hormone: *see* TESTOSTERONE.

Retcin. Antibiotic: *see* ERYTHROMYCIN.

Retin-A. Topical treatment for acne: *see* TRETINOIN.

Retinova. Topical treatment used to improve appearance of skin affected by long term exposure to sun: *see* TRETINOIN.

Retrovir. Antiviral: *see* ZIDOVUDINE.

Revanil. Dopamine agonist for use in Parkinson's disease: *see* LYSURIDE.

Rheomacrodex. Plasma expander: *see* DEXTRANS.

Rheumacin L.A. Sustained-release, non-steroid anti-inflammatory/analgesic: *see* INDOMETHACIN.

Rheumox. Non-steroid anti-inflammatory: *see* AZAPROPAZONE.

Rhinocort. Corticosteroid nasal spray for treatment of nasal symptoms, hay fever and other nasal allergies: *see* BUDESONIDE.

Rhinolast. Antihistamine nasal spray: *see* AZELASTINE.

Rhotard. Sustained release analgesic: *see* MORPHINE.

Ridaura. Orally active gold compound for treatment of rheumatoid arthritis: *see* AURANOFIN.

Rifadin. Anti-tuberculosis: *see* RIFAMPICIN.

Rifater. Anti-tuberculosis: *see* ISONIAZID, PYRAZINAMIDE, RIFAMPICIN.

Rifinah. Anti-tuberculosis: *see* ISONIAZID, RIFAMPICIN.

Rilutek. To slow the progression of motor neurone disease: *see* RILUZOLE.

Rimactane. Anti-tuberculosis: *see* RIFAMPICIN.

Rimactazid. Anti-tuberculosis: *see* ISONIAZID, RIFAMPICIN.

Rimso-50. Used in bladder inflammation: *see* DIMETHYL SULPHOXIDE.

Rinatec. Nasal spray for relief of watery nasal discharge: *see* IPRATROPIUM.

Risperdal. Antipsychotic: *see* RISPERIDONE.

Rite-Diet gluten-free (b). Dietary substitute for GLUTEN sensitivity.

Rite-Diet protein-free (b). Dietary substitute for protein intolerance (e.g., renal failure).

Rivotril. Anticonvulsant: *see* CLONAZEPAM.

Roaccutane. VITAMIN A derivative: *see* ISOTRETINOIN.

Robaxin. Muscle relaxant: *see* METHOCARBAMOL.

Robaxisal forte (d). As Robaxin 750 plus ACETYLSALICYLIC ACID.

Robinul. Anticholinergic for peptic ulcers: *see* GLYCOPYRRONIUM.

Robinul neostigmine. As Robinul with NEOSTIGMINE.

Rocaltrol. Vitamin used for correction of calcium and phosphate metabolism in renal osteodystrophy and in post menopausal osteoporosis: *see* CALCITRIOL.

Rocephin. Antibiotic: *see* CEFTRIAXONE.

Roferon-A. Antiviral agent used to treat an AIDS-associated tumour and chronic myelogenous leukaemia and chronic hepatitis C: *see* INTERFERON ALPHA-2A.

Rogitine. For diagnostic test/treatment of phaeochromocytoma: *see* PHENTOLAMINE.

Rohypnol (c). Hypnotic: *see* FLUNITRAZEPAM.

Romozin. For non-insulin dependent diabetes: *see* TROGLITAZONE.

Ronicol. Peripheral vasodilator: *see* NICOTINYL TARTRATE.

Rosoxacin. *See* ACROSOXACIN.

Roter. Antacid: *see* BISMUTH SUBNITRATE, FRANGULA, MAGNESIUM CARBONATE, SODIUM BICARBONATE.

Rotersept. Antiseptic spray for prevention of mastitis during lactation: *see* CHLORHEXIDINE.

Rowachol. For biliary disorders: *see* CAMPHOR, EUCALYPTUS, MENTHOL.

Rowatinex. For biliary disorders. Mixture of ESSENTIAL OILS (e.g., ANETHOLE, CAMPHOR, EUCALYPTUS).

Rozex. Topical antibiotic treatment for rosacea: *see* METRONIDAZOLE.

Rubavax (d). Freeze dried vaccine for active immunization against rubella. Contains low concentration of NEOMYCIN and is contraindicated if the patient is sensitive to this drug.

Rynacrom. Topical insufflation for allergic rhinitis: *see* SODIUM CROMOGLYCATE.

Rynacrom compound. As Rynacrom with XYLOMETAZOLINE.

Rythmodan. Antidysrhythmic: *see* DISOPYRAMIDE.

Rythmodan retard. Sustained-release formulation of Rythmodan.

S

Sabril. Anticonvulsant: *see* VIGABATRIN.

Saizen. Synthetic human growth hormone used to treat growth failure in children due to growth hormone deficiency: *see* SOMATROPIN.

Salactol. Topical treatment for warts: *see* LACTIC ACID, SALICYLIC ACID.

Salagen. To treat dry mouth associated with radiotherapy: *see* PILOCARPINE.

Salatac. Topical treatment for warts: *see* SALICYLIC ACID, LACTIC ACID.

Salazopyrin. For ulcerative colitis: *see* SULPHASALAZINE.

Salbulin (d). Sympathomimetic bronchodilator: *see* SALBUTAMOL.

Salofalk. For ulcerative colitis: *see* MESALAZINE.

Salonair. Rubefacient: *see* BENZYL NICOTINATE, CAMPHOR, GLYCOL SALICYLATE, MENTHOL, METHYL SALICYLATE, SQUALANE.

Saluric. Diuretic: *see* CHLOROTHIAZIDE.

Salzone. Analgesic: *see* PARACETAMOL.

Sandimmun (d). Immunosuppressant: *see* CYCLOSPORIN.

Sandocal. Effervescent supplement for calcium deficiency states.

Sandoglobulin. Concentrate of IMMUNOGLOBULIN for patients with deficiency of this protein.

Sando-K. Effervescent potassium supplement. Mixture of POTASSIUM CHLORIDE and POTASSIUM BICARBONATE. Provides potassium and chloride ions for absorption. Gastric irritation much less than with simple potassium chloride solution. Some irritation may still occur. Danger of hyperkalaemia if used in renal failure, treated by haemodialysis and ion exchange resins.

Sandostatin. For relief of symptoms of gastroenteropancreatic insulin secreting tumours and endocrine tumours, e.g. carcinoid syndrome: *see* OCTREOTIDE.

Sandrena. Hormone replacement therapy for post menopausal symptoms: *see* OESTRADIOL.

Sanomigran. Migraine prophylactic: *see* PIZOTIFEN.

Saventrine. Slow-release sympathomimetic for heart block: *see* ISOPRENALINE.

Schering PC4. Oral postcoital contraceptive: *see* ETHINYLOESTRADIOL, NORGESTREL.

Scheriproct. Topical treatment for haemorrhoids: *see* CINCHOCAINE, PREDNISOLONE.

Scoline (d). Muscle relaxant: *see* SUXAMETHONIUM.

Scopoderm TTS. Antiemetic for travel sickness. Absorbed through the skin from a self-adhesive patch: *see* HYOSCINE HYDROBROMIDE.

Secadrex. Antihypertensive: *see* ACEBUTOLOL, HYDROCHLOROTHIAZIDE.

Seconal sodium (c). Sedative/hypnotic: *see* QUINALBARBITONE.

Sectral. Beta-adrenoceptor blocker: *see* ACEBUTOLOL.

Securon. Antianginal/antihypertensive: *see* VERAPAMIL.

Securopen. Antibiotic: *see* AZLOCILLIN.

Selexid. Antibiotic: *see* PIVMECILLINAM.

Selsun (b). Shampoo for seborrhoeic dermatitis: *see* SELENIUM SULPHIDE.

Semi-Daonil. Oral hypoglycaemic: *see* GLIBENCLAMIDE.

Semitard (d). Long-acting purified pork insulin (zinc suspension): *see* INSULIN.

Semprex. Antihistamine: *see* ACRIVASTINE.

Senokot. Purgative: *see* SENNA.

Septrin. Antibacterial: *see* CO-TRIMOXAZOLE.

Serc. For Ménière's syndrome: *see* BETAHISTINE.

Serdolect. Antipsychotic: *see* SERTINDOLE.

Serenace. Tranquillizer: *see* HALOPERIDOL.

Serevent. Bronchodilator: *see* SALMETEROL.

Serophene (d). For treatment of female infertility: *see* CLOMIPHENE.

Seroquel. Antipsychotic for treatment of schizophrenia: *see* QUETIAPINE.

Seroxat. Antidepressant: *see* PAROXETINE.

Sevredol. Analgesic: *see* MORPHINE.

Simeco. Antacid: *see* ACTIVATED DIMETHICONE, ALUMINIUM HYDROXIDE, MAGNESIUM CARBONATE, MAGNESIUM HYDROXIDE.

Simplene. Eye drops for glaucoma: *see* ADRENALINE.

Sinemet preparations. Antiparkinsonian containing varying doses of LEVODOPA plus CARBIDOPA.

Sinequan. Anxiolytic/antidepressant: *see* DOXEPIN.

Singulair. Antiasthmatic: *see* MONTELUKAST.

Sinthrome. Anticoagulant: *see* NICOUMALONE.

Siopel. Soothing, antiseptic cream for skin rashes: *see* CETRIMIDE, DIMETHICONE.

Skelid. Used in Paget's disease: *see* TILUDRONIC ACID.

Skinoren. Topical treatment for acne: *see* AZELAIC ACID.

Skin testing solutions. Allergen extracts used in skin testing for allergies.

Slo-Indo. Anti-inflammatory analgesic: *see* INDOMETHACIN.

Slophyllin. Sustained-release bronchodilator: *see* THEOPHYLLINE.

Sloprolol. Sustained-release beta-adrenoceptor blocker: *see* PROPRANOLOL.

Slow-Fe. Slow-release haematinic: *see* FERROUS SULPHATE.

Slow-Fe folic. Slow-release haematinic as Slow-Fe plus FOLIC ACID.

Slow-K. Slow-release POTASSIUM CHLORIDE.

Slow-Pren. Sustained-release antihypertensive: *see* OXPRENOLOL.

Slow Sodium. Slow-release SODIUM CHLORIDE.

Slow-Trasicor. Antihypertensive. Sustained-release formulation of OXPRENOLOL.

Slozem. Sustained release antihypertensive, antianginal: *see* DILTIAZEM.

Sno Phenicol. Anti-infective eye drops: *see* CHLORAMPHENICOL.

Sno-Pilo. Miotic eye drops for glaucoma: *see* PILOCARPINE.

Sno-Pro. Milk replacement for patients with phenylketonuria.

Sno Tears. Lubricant eye drops for dry eyes: *see* POLYVINYL ALCOHOL.

Sodium Amytal (c). Hypnotic/sedative: *see* AMYLOBARBITONE.

Sofradex. Corticosteroid/anti-infective drops for use in eyes or ears: *see* DEXAMETHASONE, FRAMYCETIN, GRAMICIDIN.

Soframycin. Topical anti-infective: *see* FRAMYCETIN, GRAMICIDIN.

Soframycin inj. and tabs. Antibiotic: *see* FRAMYCETIN.

Sofra-Tulle. Gauze dressing with antimicrobial: *see* FRAMYCETIN.

Solarcaine. Local anaesthetic cream: *see* BENZOCAINE, TRICLOSAN.

Solian. Antipsychotic for treatment of schizophrenia: *see* AMISULPRIDE.

Solis. Anxiolytic: *see* DIAZEPAM.

Solivito N. Vitamins for injection: *see* ANEURINE, BIOTIN, CYANOCOBALAMIN, FOLIC ACID, NICOTINAMIDE, PANTOTHENIC ACID, PYRIDOXINE, RIBOFLAVINE, VITAMIN C.

Solpadeine. Soluble, effervescent analgesic: *see* CAFFEINE, CODEINE, PARACETAMOL.

Solpadol. Analgesic: *see* CODEINE PHOSPHATE, PARACETAMOL.

Solu-Cortef. Corticosteroid injection: *see* HYDROCORTISONE.

Solu-Medrone. Corticosteroid injection: *see* METHYLPREDNISOLONE.

Solvazinc. Soluble zinc supplements for zinc-deficiency states: *see* ZINC SULPHATE.

Somatuline. Treatment for acromegaly: *see* LANREOTIDE.

Sominex. Antihistamine hypnotic: *see* PROMETHAZINE.

Somnite. Hypnotic: *see* NITRAZEPAM.

Soneryl (c). Hypnotic/sedative: *see* BUTOBARBITONE.

Sorbichew. Antianginal, chewable tablets: *see* ISOSORBIDE DINITRATE.

Sorbid SA. Sustained-release vasodilator for prophylaxis of angina: *see* ISOSORBIDE DINITRATE.

Sorbitrate. Antianginal chewable tablets: *see* ISOSORBIDE DINITRATE.

Sotacor. Beta-adrenoceptor blocker: *see* SOTALOL.

Soya formula. Substitute for cow's milk in infant feeds. For use in intolerance to cow's milk, sucrose and lactose. Contains carbohydrate (from corn syrup), fat (from vegetable oils), and protein (from soya), together with vitamins and minerals.

Sparine (d). Tranquillizer/antiemetic: *see* PROMAZINE.

Spasmonal. Antispasmodic for gastro-intestinal or uterine spasm: *see* ALVERINE.

Spectraban (b). Topical application for protection of skin from ultraviolet light.

Spiretic. Diuretic: *see* SPIRONOLACTONE.

Spiroctan. Diuretic: *see* SPIRONOLACTONE.

Spiroctan M. Diuretic: *see* POTASSIUM CANRENOATE.

Spirolone. Diuretic: *see* SPIRONOLACTONE.

Sporanox. Oral antifungal for vulvovaginal candidiasis, pityriasis versicolor and dermatophytoses: *see* ITRACONAZOLE.

Sprilon. Soothing, protective skin cream: *see* DIMETHICONE, ZINC OXIDE.

Stafoxil. Antibiotic: *see* FLUCLOXACILLIN.

Staril. Antihypertensive: *see* FOSINOPRIL.

Staycept. Spermicidal jelly: *see* OCTOXYNOL.

STD inj. Scleroses varicose veins: *see* SODIUM TETRADECYL SULPHATE.

Stelazine. Tranquillizer: *see* TRIFLUOPERAZINE.

Stemetil. Tranquillizer/antiemetic/antivertigo: *see* PROCHLORPERAZINE.

Ster-Zac (b). Topical anti-infective: *see* HEXACHLOROPHANE.

Stesolid. Anticonvulsant: *see* DIAZEPAM.

Stiedex. Corticosteroid cream for dermatitis: *see* DESOXYMETHASONE.

Stiedex LPN. Corticosteroid/antibiotic cream for infected dermatitis: *see* DESOXYMETHASONE, NEOMYCIN.

Stiemycin. Antibiotic solution for topical application in acne: *see* ERYTHROMYCIN.

Stilnoct. Hypnotic: *see* ZOLPIDEM.

Streptase. Fibrinolytic: *see* STREPTOKINASE.

Stromba. Anabolic steroid: *see* STANOZOLOL.

Stugeron. Antiemetic/antivertigo: *see* CINNARIZINE.

Sublimaze (c). Narcotic analgesic: *see* FENTANYL.

Sudafed. Decongestant: *see* PSEUDOEPHEDRINE.

Sudafed Co. As Sudafed with PARACETAMOL.

Sudafed Expectorant. As Sudafed with GUAIPHENESIN.

Sudafed Linctus. As Sudafed with DEXTROMETHORPHAN.

Sudafed Plus. As Sudafed with TRIPROLIDINE.

Sudocrem. Bland topical cream for bed sores, nappy rash, and burns: *see* BENZYLBENZOATE, LANOLIN, ZINC OXIDE.

Suleo (b). Shampoo for head lice: *see* CARBARYL.

Suleo-M. Topical treatment for lice: *see* MALATHION.

Sulparex. Antipsychotic: *see* SULPIRIDE.

Sulpitil. Antipsychotic: *see* SULPIRIDE.

Sultrin vaginal preps. Local antibacterial combination: *see* SULPHABENZAMIDE, SULPHACETAMIDE, SULPHATHIAZOLE.

Suprax. Antibacterial: *see* CEFIXIME.

Suprecur. Clotting factor concentrate for treatment of Haemophilia B or Christmas Disease: *see* FACTOR IX.

Suprefact. Hormone: *see* BUSERELIN.

Surem. Hypnotic: *see* NITRAZEPAM.

Surgam. Non-steroid anti-inflammatory/analgesic: *see* TIAPROFENIC ACID.

Surmontil. Antidepressive: *see* TRIMIPRAMINE.

Survanta. Treatment for lung damage (Respiratory Distress Syndrome) in premature babies requiring mechanical ventilation: *see* BERACTANT.

Suscard buccal. Vasodilator tablets for buccal absorption: *see* GLYCERYL TRINITRATE.

Sustac. Antianginal: *see* GLYCERYL TRINITRATE.

Sustanon. Male sex hormone for deficiency states or inoperable breast carcinoma: *see* TESTOSTERONE.

Symmetrel. Antiparkinsonian and antiviral agent: *see* AMANTADINE.

Synacthen. Synthetic corticotrophic injection: *see* TETRACOSACTRIN.

Synalar. Corticosteroid: *see* FLUOCINOLONE.

Synalar C and N. Topical corticosteroid/anti-infective: *see* CLIOQUINOL, FLUOCINOLONE, NEOMYCIN.

Synarel. Synthetic hormone tor intranasal treatment of endometriosis: *see* NAFARELIN.

Syndol. Analgesic: *see* CAFFEINE, CODEINE, DOXYLAMINE, PARACETAMOL.

Synflex. Non-steroid anti-inflammatory/ analgesic: *see* NAPROXEN.

Synphase. Oral contraceptive: *see* ETHINYLOESTRADIOL, NORETHISTERONE.

Syntaris. Topical corticosteroid spray for nasal allergies: *see* FLUNISOLIDE.

Synthamin. AMINO ACIDS and electrolyte sources for intravenous feeding.

Synthamix. Amino acids, glucose and electrolytes for parenteral nutrition.

Syntocinon. Synthetic pituitary hormone: *see* OXYTOCIN.

Syntometrine. Contracts uterine muscle: *see* ERGOMETRINE, OXYTOCIN.

Syntopressin. Synthetic pituitary hormone: *see* LYPRESSIN.

Syscor MR. Antianginal, antihypertensive: *see* NISOLDIPINE.

Sytron. For iron-deficiency anaemia: *see* SODIUM IRON EDETATE.

T

Tagamet. Gastric histamine receptor blocker; reduces acid secretion: *see* CIMETIDINE.

Tambocor. Antiarrhythmic: *see* FLECAINIDE.

Tamofen. For treatment of anovular infertility and breast cancer: *see* TAMOXIFEN.

Tampovagan. Pessaries containing STILBOESTROL or NEOMYCIN for vaginal complaints.

Tancolin. Cough suppressant: *see* DEXTROMETHORPHAN.

Tarband. Zinc and COAL TAR bandage for eczema.

Tarcortin. Corticosteroid cream: *see* COAL TAR, HYDROCORTISONE.

Targocid. Antibiotic: *see* TEICOPLANIN.

Tarivid. Antibacterial: *see* OFLOXACIN.

Tarka. Antihypertensive: *see* TRANDOLAPRIL, VERAPAMIL.

Tasmar. For Parkinson's disease: *see* TOLCAPONE.

Tavanic. Antibiotic: *see* LEVOFLOXACIN.

Tavegil. Antihistamine: *see* CLEMASTINE.

Taxol. Cytotoxic: *see* PACLITAXEL.

Taxotere. Cytotoxic to treat breast cancer: *see* DOCETAXEL.

Tazocin. Antibiotic: *see* PIPERACILLIN.

Tears Naturale. Drops for dry eyes: *see* DEXTRANS, HYPROMELLOSE.

Teejel. Gel for application to gums in dental pain: *see* CHOLINE SALICYLATE, CETALKONIUM.

Tegretol. Anticonvulsant: *see* CARBAMAZEPINE.

Telfast. Antihistamine: *see* FEXOFENADINE.

Temgesic (c). Analgesic: *see* BUPRENORPHINE.

Temopen (d). Antibiotic: *see* TEMOCILLIN.

Tenben. Antihypertensive: *see* ATENOLOL, BENDROFLUAZIDE.

Tenif. Antihypertensive: *see* ATENOLOL, NIFEDIPINE.

Tenoret-50. Antihypertensive: *see* ATENOLOL, CHLORTHALIDONE.

Tenoretic. Antihypertensive combination identical to Tenoret-50 but double dose of both drugs.

Tenormin. Beta-adrenoceptor blocker: *see* ATENOLOL.

Tensilon. Diagnostic for myasthenia gravis: *see* EDROPHONIUM.

Tensium. Anxiolytic: *see* DIAZEPAM.

Teoptic. Eye drops for glaucoma: *see* CARTEOLOL.

Terolin. Smooth muscle bladder relaxant to reduce urinary frequency: *see* TERODILINE.

Terpoin. Cough suppressant: *see* CODEINE, ESSENTIAL OILS.

Terra-Cortril. Antibiotic/corticosteroid: *see* HYDROCORTISONE, OXYTETRACYCLINE, POLYMYXIN B.

Terra-Cortril Nystatin. Antibiotic/ corticosteroid: *see* HYDROCORTISONE, NYSTATIN, OXYTETRACYCLINE.

Terramycin. Antibiotic: *see* OXYTETRACYCLINE.

Tertroxin. Thyroid hormone: *see* LIOTHYRONINE.

Tetrachel. Antibiotic: *see* TETRACYCLINE.

Tetralysal. Antibiotic: *see* LYMECYCLINE.

T-Gel. Shampoo for psoriasis, dandruff, eczema: *see* COAL TAR.

Theo-dur. Sustained-release bronchodilator: *see* THEOPHYLLINE.

Thephorin. Antihistamine: *see* PHENINDAMINE.

Thovaline. Skin protective: *see* ZINC OXIDE.

Tiempe. Antibiotic: *see* TRIMETHOPRIM.

Tilade. Aerosol inhalation for preventive treatment of asthma and bronchitis with reversible obstruction of the airways: *see* NEDOCROMIL.

Tildiem. Antianginal and antihypertensive: *see* DILTIAZEM.

Timentin. Antibacterial: *see* CLAVULANIC ACID, TICARCILLIN.

Timodine. Antifungal/corticosteroid cream: *see* BENZALKONIUM, DIMETHICONE, HYDROCORTISONE, NYSTATIN.

Timoptol. Eye drops for glaucoma: *see* TIMOLOL.

Tinaderm M. Topical antifungal: *see* NYSTATIN, TOLNAFTATE.

Tisept. Topical disinfectant: *see* CETRIMIDE, CHLORHEXIDINE.

Titralac. Antacid: *see* CALCIUM CARBONATE.

Tixylix. Cough suppressant mixture: *see* PHOLCODINE, PROMETHAZINE.

Tobralex (d). Antibiotic: *see* TOBRAMYCIN.

Tofranil. Antidepressant: *see* IMIPRAMINE.

Tolanase. Oral hypoglycaemic: *see* TOLAZAMIDE.

Tolectin (d). Non-steroid anti-inflammatory/ analgesic: *see* TOLMETIN.

Tomudex. Cytotoxic for treatment of large bowel cancer: *see* RALTITREXED.

Tonocard (d). Antiarrhythmic: *see* TOCAINIDE.

Topal. Antacid: *see* ALGINIC ACID, ALUMINIUM HYDROXIDE, MAGNESIUM CARBONATE.

Topamax. Anticonvulsant: *see* TOPIRAMATE.

Topicycline. Antibiotic for topical application in acne: *see* TETRACYCLINE.

Toradol. Non-steroidal anti-inflammatory analgesic for post-operative pain: *see* KETOROLAC.

Torbetol. Topical antibacterial for acne: *see* BENZALKONIUM, CETRIMIDE, HEXACHLOROPHANE.

Torem. Diuretic: *see* TORASEMIDE.

Tracrium. Muscle relaxant: *see* ATRACURIUM.

Tramake Insts. Analgesic: *see* TRAMADOL.

Trandate. Antihypertensive: *see* LABETALOL.

Transiderm-Nitro. Transdermal preparation for prophylactic treatment of angina pectoris whereby the drug is applied to the skin on a self-adhesive patch: *see* GLYCERYL TRINITRATE.

Transvasin. Rubefacient: *see* BENZOCAINE, ETHYL NICOTINATE, SALICYLIC ACID.

Tranxene. Tranquillizer: *see* CLORAZEPATE.

Trasicor. Beta-adrenoceptor blocker: *see* OXPRENOLOL.

Trasidrex. Antihypertensive: *see* CYCLOPENTHIAZIDE, OXPRENOLOL.

Trasylol. Used in acute pancreatitis: *see* APROTININ.

Travasept. Disinfectant: *see* CETRIMIDE, CHLORHEXIDINE.

Travasept 30. Topical disinfectant to be used undiluted for wound and skin disinfection: *see* CETRIMIDE, CHLORHEXIDINE.

Travogyn. For treatment of vaginal infections: *see* ISOCONAZOLE.

Traxam. Fibrinolytic: *see* FELBINAC.

Trental. Peripheral vasodilator: *see* OXPENTIFYLLINE.

Treosulfan. Cytotoxic: *see* THREITOL DIMETHANE SULPHONATE.

TRH. Hormone: *see* PROTIRELIN.

Tri-Adcortyl. Topical corticosteroid/antibiotic: *see* GRAMICIDIN, NEOMYCIN, NYSTATIN, TRIAMCINOLONE.

Triadene. Oral contraceptive: *see* ETHINYLOESTRADIOL, GESTODENE.

Triamco. Diuretic: *see* HYDROCHLOROTHIAZIDE, TRIAMTERENE.

Tridestra. Sex hormones for post-menopausal symptoms: *see* MEDROXYPROGESTERONE, OESTRADIOL.

Triludan. Antihistamine: *see* TERFENADINE.

Trimogal. Antimicrobial: *see* TRIMETHOPRIM.

Trimopan. Antimicrobial: *see* TRIMETHOPRIM.

Trimovate. Topical corticosteroid/anti-infective: *see* CLOBETASONE, NYSTATIN, OXYTETRACYCLINE.

Trinordiol. Oral contraceptive: *see* ETHINYLOESTRADIOL, LEVONORGESTREL.

TriNovum. Oral contraceptive with three different strengths for use at different stages of the menstrual cycle: *see* ETHINYLOESTRADIOL, NORETHISTERONE.

Triperidol. Antipsychotic: *see* TRIFLUPERIDOL.

Triptafen M. Antidepressant/ tranquillizer: *see* AMITRIPTYLINE, PERPHENAZINE.

Trisequens. Female sex hormones for menopausal symptoms: *see* NORETHISTERONE, OESTRADIOL.

Tritace. Antihypertensive: *see* RAMIPRIL.

Trivax. Triple vaccination against diphtheria, tetanus, and pertussis.

Trobicin. Long-acting, single-dose antibiotic for gonorrhoea: *see* SPECTINOMYCIN.

Tropergen. Antidiarrhoeal: *see* ATROPINE SULPHATE, DIPHENOXYLATE.

Tropium. Anxiolytic: *see* CHLORDIAZEPOXIDE.

Trosyl. Topical antifungal for nail infections: *see* TICONAZOLE.

Trusopt. Topical treatment for glaucoma: *see* DORZOLAMIDE.

Tryptizol. Tricyclic antidepressant: *see* AMITRIPTYLINE.

Tuberculin Tine Test. Intradermal injection test for tuberculosis: *see* TUBERCULIN.

Tuinal (c). Hypnotic: *see* AMYLOBARBITONE, QUINALBARBITONE.

Twinrix. Combined vaccine for hepatitis A and hepatitis B.

Tylex. Analgesic: *see* CODEINE, PARACETAMOL.

Typhim Vi. Vaccine: *see* TYPHOID VACCINE.

Tyrozets. Local anaesthetic throat lozenges: *see* BENZOCAINE, TYROTHRICIN.

U V

Ubretid. Anticholinesterase: *see* DISTIGMINE.

Ukidan. Fibrinolytic injection: *see* UROKINASE.

Ultiva. Analgesic for use in general anaesthesia: *see* REMIFENTANIL.

Ultrabase. Bland, protective cream recommended for use when topical steroids are withdrawn: *see* LIQUID PARAFFIN, SOFT PARAFFIN, STEARYL ALCOHOL.

Ultralanum. Topical corticosteroid/anti-infective: *see* CLEMIZOLE, FLUOCORTOLONE.

Ultraproct. Local treatment for haemorrhoids: *see* CINCHOCAINE, FLUOCORTOLONE.

Ultratard. Long-acting purified beef insulin (zinc suspension): *see* INSULIN.

Unguentum. Protective cream for use on skin. May be used as vehicle for drugs.

Uniflu. For symptomatic treatment of common cold: *see* CAFFEINE, CODEINE, DIPHENHYDRAMINE, PARACETAMOL, PHENYLEPHRINE, VITAMIN C.

Unigest. Antacid: *see* ALUMINIUM HYDROXIDE, DIMETHICONE.

Unihep. Anticoagulant: *see* HEPARIN.

Uniparin. Anticoagulant for subcutaneous injection: *see* HEPARIN.

Uniphyllin. Sustained-release bronchodilator: *see* THEOPHYLLINE.

Uniroid. Local treatment for haemorrhoids: *see* CINCHOCAINE, HYDROCORTISONE, NEOMYCIN, POLYMIX B.

Unisept. Topical disinfectant: *see* CHLORHEXIDINE.

Unisomnia. Hypnotic: *see* NITRAZEPAM.

Univer. Antianginal/antihypertensive: *see* VERAPAMIL.

Urdox. Bile acid for dissolution of cholesterol gall stones: *see* URSODEOXYCHOLIC ACID.

Uriben. Antibiotic: *see* NALIDIXIC ACID.

Urispas. Anticholinergic antispasmodic for urinary tract colic: *see* FLAVOXATE.

Uromitexan. Used to prevent bladder toxicity resulting from cyclophosphamide treatment: *see* CYCLOPHOSPHAMIDE, MESNA.

Uro-Tainer. Sterile solution for maintenance of urinary catheters: *see* CHLORHEXIDINE, MAGNESIUM CITRATE, MANDELIC ACID, SODIUM CHLORIDE.

Ursofalk. Bile acid for dissolution of cholesterol gall stones: *see* URSODEOXYCHOLIC ACID.

Utinor. Antibacterial: *see* NORFLOXACIN.

Utovlan. Hormone: *see* NORETHISTERONE.

Uvistat (b). Topical applications for protection of skin from ultraviolet light: *see* MEXENONE.

Vagifem. Hormone for vaginal application in menopausal conditions: *see* OESTRADIOL.

Valium. Anxiolytic: *see* DIAZEPAM.

Vallergan. Antihistamine: *see* TRIMEPRAZINE.

Valoid. Antihistamine: *see* CYCLIZINE.

Valtrex. Antiviral: *see* VALACICLOVIR.

Vamin. Amino acids and carbohydrate for intravenous nutrition.

Vancocin. Antibiotic: *see* VANCOMYCIN.

Vansil. Antischistosomiasis: *see* OXAMNIQUINE.

Varidase. Enzymes for topical use in the removal of fibrinous or blood clots: *see* STREPTODORNASE, STREPTOKINASE.

Varihesive. Impregnated bandage: *see* CARMELLOSE, GELATIN, PECTIN.

Vascace. Antihypertensive: *see* CILAZAPRIL.

Vasogen. Soothing, protective cream for sore skin: *see* CALAMINE, DIMETHICONE, ZINC OXIDE.

Vasoxine. Vasoconstrictor: *see* METHOXAMINE.

Vectavir. Topical antiviral: *see* PENCICLOVIR.

Veganin. Analgesic: *see* ACETYLSALICYLIC ACID, CODEINE, PARACETAMOL.

Velbe. Cytotoxic: *see* VINBLASTINE.

Velosef. Antibiotic: *see* CEPHRADINE.

Velosulin. Purified crystalline pork insulin: *see* INSULIN.

Ventide. Sympathomimetic/steroid aerosol for asthma: *see* BECLOMETHASONE, SALBUTAMOL.

Ventmax. Sustained release bronchodilator: *see* SALBUTAMOL

Ventodisks. Inhalation system for bronchodilation: *see* SALBUTAMOL.

Ventolin. Sympathomimetic bronchodilator: *see* SALBUTAMOL.

Vepesid. Cytotoxic: *see* ETOPOSIDE.

Veractil. Antipsychotic: *see* METHOTRIMEPRAZINE.

Veracur. Topical treatment for warts: *see* FORMALDEHYDE.

Veripaque. Laxative: *see* OXYPHENISATIN.

Verkade (b). GLUTEN-free biscuits for gluten-sensitive bowel disorders.

Vermox. For threadworms, whipworms, roundworms, hookworms: *see* MEBENDAZOLE.

Verrugon. Ointment for warts: *see* SALICYLIC ACID.

Verucasep. For treatment of warts: *see* GLUTARALDEHYDE.

Vesanoid. Used with chemotherapy in treatment of leukaemia: *see* TRETINOIN.

Viazem XL. Sustained release antianginal/antihypertensive: *see* DILTIAZEM.

Vibramycin. Antibiotic: *see* DOXYCYCLINE.

Vibramycin-D. Water-dispersible antibiotic tablets, avoids the danger of oesophageal damage which may occur with capsules: *see* DOXYCYCLINE.

Videne (d). Disinfectant: *see* POVIDONE-IODINE.

Videx. Antiviral for use in advanced AIDS: *see* DIDANOSINE.

Vidopen. Antibiotic: *see* AMPICILLIN.

Vigranon B. Vitamin syrup: *see* ANEURINE, NICOTINAMIDE, PANTHENOL, PYRIDOXINE, RIBOFLAVINE.

Vioform-Hydrocortisone. Topical anti-infective: *see* CLOQUINOL, HYDROCORTISONE.

Viracept. Antiviral for use in HIV positive patients with evidence of immunodeficiency: *see* NELFINAVIR.

Viraferon. Treatment for hepatitis B and C: *see* INTERFERON ALPHA-2B.

Viramune. Antiviral for use in HIV positive patients with evidence of immunodeficiency: *see* NEVIRAPINE.

Virazid. Antiviral: *see* RIBAVIRIN.

Virormone. Hormone injection: *see* TESTOSTERONE.

Visclair. Reduces mucous viscosity: *see* METHYLCYSTEINE.

Viscopaste. Impregnated bandage: *see* ZINC OXIDE.

Viscotears. Tear substitute: *see* POLYACRYLIC ACID.

Viskaldix. Antihypertensive: *see* CLOPAMIDE, PINDOLOL.

Visken. Beta-adrenoceptor blocker: *see* PINDOLOL.

Vista-Methasone N. Corticosteroid/antibiotic nasal drops: *see* BETAMETHASONE, NEOMYCIN.

Vistide. Antiviral: *see* CIDOFOVIR.

Vitlipid. Fat-soluble vitamins for parenteral nutrition with fat solutions: *see* CALCIFEROL, PHYTOMENADIONE, VITAMIN A.

Vivalan. Antidepressant: *see* VILOXAZINE.

Vivapryl. Used to treat Parkinson's disease: *see* SELEGILINE.

Vividrin. For prevention and treatment of allergic conjunctivitis: *see* SODIUM CROMOGLYCATE.

Vivotif. Oral vaccine: *see* TYPHOID VACCINE.

Volmax. Sustained-release bronchodilator: *see* SALBUTAMOL.

Volsaid Retard. Sustained release anti-inflammatory: *see* DICLOFENAC.

Voltarol. Non-steroid anti-inflammatory/analgesic: *see* DICLOFENAC.

Voltarol Emugel. Topical non-steroidal anti-inflammatory/analgesic: *see* DICLOFENAC.

Voltarol ophtha. Eye drops for use after cataract surgery: *see* DICLOFENAC.

W X Y Z

Warticon. Topical treatment for genital warts: *see* PODOPHYLLOTOXIN.

Waxsol. Drops to soften ear wax: *see* DIOCTYL SODIUM SULPHOSUCCINATE.

Welldorm. Hypnotic: *see* CHLORAL BETAINE.

Wellferon. For treatment of 'hairy cell' leukaemia: *see* INTERFERON ALPHA-NI.

Wellvone. Antiprotozoal: *see* ATOVAQUONE.

Wright's vaporizer. Inhalation for nasal, bronchial congestion: *see* CHLOROCRESOL.

Xalatan. Eyedrops for treatment of glaucoma: *see* LATANOPROST.

Xanax. Anxiolytic: *see* ALPRAZOLAM.

Xatral. $Alpha_1$ antagonist used for symptomatic treatment of benign prostatic hypertrophy: *see* ALFUZOSIN.

X-Prep. Preradiography purgative: *see* SENNA.

Xylocaine. Local anaesthetic: *see* LIGNOCAINE.

Xylocard. Antiarrhythmic: *see* LIGNOCAINE.

Xyloproct. Local anaesthetic/ corticosteroid for anal conditions: *see* HYDROCORTISONE, LIGNOCAINE, ZINC OXIDE.

Xylotox preps. Local anaesthetic: *see* ADRENALINE, LIGNOCAINE.

Yomesan. For tapeworms: *see* NICLOSAMIDE.

Yutopar. Uterine relaxant: *see* RITODRINE.

Zacin. Topical analgesic cream for use in osteoarthritis: *see* CAPSAICIN.

Zaditen. Antihistamine for prevention of asthma: *see* KETOTIFEN.

Zamadol. Analgesic for moderate to severe pain: *see* TRAMADOL.

Zanaflex. Muscle relaxant: *see* TIZANIDINE.

Zanidip. Antihypertensive: *see* LERCANIDIPINE.

Zantac. Gastric histamine receptor blocker. Reduces acid secretion: *see* RANITIDINE.

Zarontin. Anti-epileptic: *see* ETHOSUXIMIDE.

Zavedos. Cytotoxic antibiotic used to treat leukaemia: *see* IDARUBICIN.

Zeasorb. Powder for excessive perspiration: *see* CHLOROXYLENOL.

Zerit. Antiviral for treatment of HIV infection: *see* STAVUDINE.

Zestoretic. Antihypertensive: *see* HYDROCHLOROTHIAZIDE, LISINOPRIL.

Zestril. Antihypertensive: *see* LISINOPRIL.

Zidoval. Antibacterial: *see* METRONIDAZOLE.

Zimovane. Hypnotic for insomnia: *see* ZOPICLONE.

Zinacef. Antibiotic: *see* CEFUROXIME.

Zinamide. Anti-tuberculosis: *see* PYRAZINAMIDE.

Zincaband. Zinc paste bandage.

Zincomed. For zinc deficiency: *see* ZINC SULPHATE.

Zineryt. Topical antibiotic for treatment of acne: *see* ERYTHROMYCIN, ZINC ACETATE.

Zinga. Gastric histamine receptor blocker; reduces acid secretion: *see* NIZATIDINE.

Zinnat. Antibiotic: *see* CEFUROXIME.

Zirtek. Antihistamine: *see* CETIRIZINE DIHYDROCHLORIDE.

Zispin. Antidepressant: *see* MIRTAZAPINE.

Zithromax. Antibiotic: *see* AZITHROMYCIN.

Zocor. For hypercholesterolaemia: *see* SIMVASTATIN.

Zofran. Antiemetic for treatment of vomiting caused by cytotoxic chemotherapy, radiotherapy and surgery: *see* ONDANSETRON.

Zoladex. Hormone for treatment of cancer of the prostate gland, breast cancer and endometriosis: *see* GOSERELIN.

Zomig. For acute migraine: *see* ZOLMITRIPTAN.

Zomoctan. Synthetic human growth hormone used to treat growth failure in children due to growth hormone deficiency: *see* SOMATROPIN.

Zomorph. Sustained release analgesic: *see* MORPHINE.

Zonulysin. For cataract extraction: *see* CHYMOTRYPSIN.

Zorac. Topical treatment for psoriasis. *see* TAZAROTENE.

Zoton. For peptic ulcers, acid-related indigestion and oesophageal reflux: *see* LANSOPRAZOLE.

Zovirax. Antiviral: *see* ACYCLOVIR.

Z Span Spansule. Sustained-release zinc for zinc deficiency: *see* ZINC SULPHATE.

Zumenon. For relief of menopausal symptoms: *see* OESTRADIOL.

Zydol. Analgesic: *see* TRAMADOL.

Zyloric. For gout: *see* ALLOPURINOL.

Zyprexa. Antipsychotic: *see* OLANZAPINE.

APPENDIX
Common slang names for misused drugs

This list of names has been compiled from several sources. Please note that the information given here cannot be as accurate as that provided elsewhere in the *Drugs Handbook,* because slang names change according to fashion. Some slang names refer to preparations that are mixtures of drugs. When names may be used to refer to one individual drug or another, rather than a mixture, the drugs are listed as alternatives (e.g. CANNABIS *or* COCAINE).

A. *see* AMPHETAMINE

Acapulco. *see* CANNABIS

Ace. *see* AMPHETAMINE *or* CANNABIS

Acid. *see* LSD *or* MDMA

Adam. *see* MDMA

Adam & Eve. *see* MDA *or* MDEA

Afghan. *see* CANNABIS

Afghan black. *see* CANNABIS

African bush. *see* CANNABIS

Amph. *see* AMPHETAMINE

Amphets. *see* AMPHETAMINE

Angels. *see* AMYLOBARBITONE *or* AMYL NITRITE

Angel dust. *see* PHENCYCLIDINE

Bananas. *see* LSD

Barbs. *see* Barbiturates *e.g.* AMYLOBARBITONE

Base. *see* COCAINE

Beam me up Scotty. *see* COCAINE, PHENCYCLIDINE (mix)

Bernice. *see* COCAINE

Bhang. *see* CANNABIS

Big brownies. *see* MDMA

Big C. *see* COCAINE

Big H. *see* HEROIN

Billy. *see* AMPHETAMINE

Billy Whizz. *see* AMPHETAMINE

Birds. *see* AMYLOBARBITONE

Biscuits. *see* MDMA

Black. *see* CANNABIS

Black and whites. *see* AMPHETAMINE *or* MDMA

Black beauties. *see* AMPHETAMINE, DEXAMPHETAMINE (DUROPHET)

Black bomber. *see* AMPHETAMINE

Black busters. *see* Barbiturates *e.g.* AMYLOBARBITONE

Black gum. *see* HEROIN

Black lightening. *see* LSD

Black pearls. *see* DIAZEPAM

Black rings. *see* LSD

Black rock. *see* AMPHETAMINE *or* CANNABIS *or* COCAINE

Black Russian. *see* CANNABIS

Black stuff. *see* OPIUM

Black tar. *see* HEROIN

Blackbirds. *see* AMPHETAMINE

Blockers. *see* Barbiturates *e.g.* AMYLOBARBITONE

Blotter. *see* LSD

Blow. *see* CANNABIS *or* COCAINE

Blue bullets. *see* Barbiturates *e.g.* AMYLOBARBITONE

Blue devils. *see* Barbiturates *e.g.* AMYLOBARBITONE

Blue dolls. *see* Barbiturates *e.g.* AMYLOBARBITONE

Blue heaven. *see* AMYLOBARBITONE *or* AMYL NITRATE

Blue star. *see* LSD

Blue unicorn. *see* LSD

Bluebirds. *see* Barbiturates *e.g.* AMYLOBARBITONE

Blues. *see* AMPHETAMINE, DEXAMPHETAMINE (DUROPHET) *or* DIETHYLPROPION

Bomber. *see* CANNABIS

Bombido. *see* AMPHETAMINE

Boo. *see* CANNABIS

Boy. *see* HEROIN

Brass. *see* CANNABIS

Brick. *see* CANNABIS

Broccoli. *see* CANNABIS

Brown. *see* HEROIN

Brown sugar. *see* HEROIN

Brown tar. *see* HEROIN

Brownies. *see* MDMA

Bubblegum. *see* CANNABIS *or* COCAINE

Burgers. *see* MDMA

Bush. *see* CANNABIS

C. *see* COCAINE

California sunrise. *see* AMPHETAMINE *or* CAFFEINE

Californian sunshine. *see* LSD *or* MDMA

Candy. *see* COCAINE *or* HEROIN *or* Barbiturates *e.g.* AMYLOBARBITONE

Carrie. *see* COCAINE

Cartwheels. *see* AMPHETAMINE

Cecil. *see* COCAINE

Charas. *see* CANNABIS

Charge. *see* CANNABIS

Chalk. *see* AMPHETAMINE

Charlie. *see* COCAINE

Chewies. *see* AMYLOBARBITONE, QUINALBARBITONE (TUINAL)

Chi. *see* HEROIN

China white. *see* FENTANYL *or* HEROIN

China whites. *see* MDA

Chinese H. *see* HEROIN

Chinese reds. *see* HEROIN

Chitari. *see* CANNABIS

Chocolate. *see* HEROIN

Cholly. *see* COCAINE

Cities. *see* MDMA

Clarity. *see* MDMA

Cloud 9. *see* COCAINE

Cocoa. *see* HEROIN

Coke. *see* COCAINE

Co-pilots. *see* AMPHETAMINE

Colombian. *see* CANNABIS

Corine. *see* COCAINE

Crack. *see* COCAINE

Crap. *see* HEROIN

Crystal. *see* COCAINE *or* METHAMPHETAMINE *or* PHENCYCLIDINE

Crystals. *see* AMPHETAMINE

Dagga (Dhaga). *see* CANNABIS

Dennis the Menace. *see* MDMA

Dexies. *see* DEXAMPHETAMINE (DEXEDRINE)

DF's. *see* DIHYDROCODEINE

Diet pills. *see* AMPHETAMINE

Dike. *see* DICONAL

Dirt. *see* HEROIN

Dirty. *see* CANNABIS

Disco biscuits. *see* MDMA

Doctor. *see* MDMA

Dog vitamins. *see* DIAZEPAM

Dog food. *see* HEROIN

Dollies. *see* METHADONE

Dolls. *see* METHADONE *or* Barbiturates *e.g.* AMYLOBARBITONE

Dominoes. *see* AMPHETAMINE, DEXAMPHETAMINE (DUROPHET)

Dope. *see* CANNABIS

Dots. *see* LSD

Double Cross. *see* AMPHETAMINE

Double Dreads. *see* AMPHETAMINE, LSD (mix)

Double 'O's. *see* MORPHINE

Double Trouble. *see* AMYLOBARBITONE, QUINALBARBITONE (TUINAL)

Double Zero. *see* CANNABIS

Dove. *see* MDMA

Downers. *see* Barbiturates *e.g.* AMYLOBARBITONE

Dragon. *see* HEROIN

Draw. *see* CANNABIS

Dream. *see* COCAINE

Dummy dust. *see* CAFFEINE, EPHEDRINE, METHAMPHETAMINE (mix)

Dust. *see* COCAINE *or* HEROIN *or* PHENCYCLIDINE

Dynamite. *see* COCAINE, MORPHINE (mix)

E. *see* MDMA *or* CANNABIS

Ecstasy. *see* MDMA

Elephant. *see* HEROIN

Essence. *see* MDMA

Eye openers. *see* AMPHETAMINE

Fantasia. *see* MDMA

Fantasy. *see* LSD, MDMA (mix) *or* LSD, MESCALINE (mix)

Fast. *see* AMPHETAMINE

Flake. *see* COCAINE

Flash. *see* LSD

Flatliners. *see* MDMA

Freebase. *see* COCAINE

French blues. *see* AMPHETAMINE

Ganja. *see* CANNABIS

Girl. *see* COCAINE

Glass. *see* METHAMPHETAMINE

Gold dust. *see* COCAINE

Gold star. *see* COCAINE

Golden haze. *see* CANNABIS

Goofballs. *see* AMPHETAMINE *or* Barbiturates *e.g.* AMYLOBARBITONE

Grass. *see* CANNABIS

Grey biscuits. *see* MDMA

Gum. *see* OPIUM *or* HEROIN

H. *see* HEROIN *or* CANNABIS

Happy dust. *see* COCAINE

Hard stuff. *see* MORPHINE

Harry. *see* HEROIN

Hash. *see* CANNABIS

Hay. *see* CANNABIS

Haze. *see* LSD

Hearts. *see* AMPHETAMINE

Heaven dust. *see* COCAINE

Hemp. *see* CANNABIS

Herb. *see* CANNABIS

Horse. *see* HEROIN *or* CANNABIS

Ice. *see* COCAINE *or* METHAMPHETAMINE

Idiot pills. *see* Barbiturates *e.g.* AMYLOBARBITONE

Jack. *see* HEROIN

Jam/Jelly. *see* COCAINE

Jane. *see* CANNABIS

Jellies. *see* TEMAZEPAM

Jelly beans. *see* AMPHETAMINE *or* TEMAZEPAM

Joint. *see* CANNABIS

Joy. *see* HEROIN

Junk. *see* DIAMORPHINE

K. *see* KETAMINE

Kermits. *see* MDMA

Kief. *see* CANNABIS

Kif. *see* CANNABIS

King Kong pills. *see* Barbiturates *e.g.* AMYLOBARBITONE

King's habit. *see* COCAINE

Kit kat. *see* KETAMINE

Knife. *see* LSD

L. *see* LSD

Lady. *see* COCAINE

Lebanese. *see* CANNABIS

Leaf. *see* CANNABIS

Liberty cap. *see* PSILOCYBIN

Lightning. *see* AMPHETAMINE

Lightning flash. *see* LSD

Liquid E. *see* KETAMINE

Liquid gold. *see* AMYL NITRITE

Liquid red. *see* AMPHETAMINE

Locker room. *see* AMYL NITRITE

Loco weed. *see* CANNABIS

Love doves. *see* MDMA

Love drug. *see* MDA *or* MDMA *or* METHAQUALONE

Love pills. *see* METHAQUALONE

Love weed. *see* CANNABIS

M & Ms. *see* MDMA

M25s. *see* MDMA

Magic mushrooms. *see* PSILOCYBIN

Malawi grass. *see* CANNABIS

Man Uniteds. *see* MDMA

Mandies. *see* METHAQUALONE (MANDRAX)

Marijuana. *see* CANNABIS

Marshmallow. *see* Barbiturates *e.g.* AMYLOBARBITONE

Mary Jane. *see* AMPHETAMINE or CANNABIS

Mary. *see* CANNABIS

Mescal. *see* MESCALINE

Meth. *see* METHADONE *or* METHAMPHETAMINE

Mexican brown. *see* HEROIN

Mexican green. *see* CANNABIS

Mexican Lebanese gold. *see* CANNABIS

Mexican mud. *see* HEROIN

Mexican reds. *see* Barbiturates *e.g.* AMYLOBARBITONE

Micro dot. *see* LSD

Mind, Body and Soul. *see* LSD

Miss Emma. *see* MORPHINE

Misties. *see* MORPHINE

Moggies. *see* NITRAZEPAM (MOGADON)

Monkey. *see* MORPHINE

Morf. *see* MORPHINE

Moroccan. *see* CANNABIS

Mosaic. *see* LSD

Mushies. *see* PSILOCYBIN

Neb. *see* Barbiturates *e.g.* AMYLOBARBITONE

Nemmies. *see* Barbiturates *e.g* AMYLOBARBITONE

Nepalese. *see* CANNABIS

New Yorkers. *see* MDMA

Nimbies. *see* Barbiturates *e.g.* AMYLOBARBITONE

Northern lights. *see* CANNABIS

Nose candy. *see* COCAINE

Nuggets. *see* COCAINE *or* AMPHETAMINE

Nutties. *see* MDMA

O. *see* OPIUM

Orange roughies. *see* MORPHINE

Orange sunshine. *see* LSD

Oranges. *see* AMPHETAMINE *or* DEXAMPHETAMINE *or* MORPHINE

Paki black. *see* CANNABIS

Palf. *see* DEXTROMORAMIDE (PALFIUM)

Panama red. *see* CANNABIS

Paper mushrooms. *see* LSD

Parachute. *see* COCAINE, HEROIN (mix)

Paradise. *see* COCAINE

PCP. *see* PHENCYCLIDINE

Peace pill. *see* PHENCYCLIDINE

Peach. *see* PALFIUM

Peanut. *see* HEROIN

Peanuts. *see* Barbiturates *e.g.* AMYLOBARBITONE

Penguins. *see* LSD

Pep pills. *see* AMPHETAMINES

Persian white. *see* HEROIN

Peter Pan. *see* MDMA *or* PHENCYCLIDINE

Phase 4, Phase 5, Phase 7. *see* MDMA

Phyamps. *see* METHADONE

Pink ladies. *see* Barbiturates *e.g.* AMYLOBARBITONE

Pinks. *see* QUINALBARBITONE

Poor man's cocaine. *see* AMPHETAMINE

Poppers. *see* AMYL NITRITE

Pot. *see* CANNABIS

Powder. *see* HEROIN *or* AMPHETAMINE

Power pack. *see* MDMA

Puff. *see* CANNABIS

Purple haze. *see* CANNABIS *or* LSD

Purple hearts. *see* DEXAMPHETAMINE

Quick. *see* KETAMINE

Rainbows. *see* LSD *or* AMYLOBARBITONE, QUINALBARBITONE (TUINAL)

Ram. *see* AMYL NITRITE

Red and whites. *see* MDMA

Red devil. *see* AMPHETAMINE *or* CAFFEINE *or* MDEA *or* PSEUDOEPHEDRINE

Red devils. *see* Barbiturates *e.g.* AMYLOBARBITONE *or* AMPHETAMINE

Red rock. *see* METHADONE

Red seal. *see* CANNABIS

Reds/Red birds. *see* Barbiturates *e.g.* AMYLOBARBITONE

Reds and blues. *see* AMYLOBARBITONE, QUINALBARBITONE (TUINAL)

Reefer. *see* CANNABIS

Resin. *see* CANNABIS

Rhubarb & Custard. *see* MDMA

Rocks. *see* COCAINE

Rocky. *see* CANNABIS

Rope. *see* CANNABIS

Rush. *see* AMYL NITRITE

Scag. *see* HEROIN

Scat. *see* HEROIN

Scooby-snack. *see* MDMA

Seggy. *see* QUINALBARBITONE (SECONAL)

Shamrocks. *see* MDMA *or* MDEA

Shrooms. *see* PSILOCYBIN

Silver Haze. *see* CANNABIS

Silver Pearl. *see* CANNABIS

Sinsemilla. *see* CANNABIS

Skag. *see* DIAMORPHINE

Skunk. *see* CANNABIS

Sleepers. *see* Barbiturates *e.g.* AMYLOBARBITONE

Sleigh-ride. *see* COCAINE

Smack. *see* DIAMORPHINE *or* COCAINE

Smilies. *see* LSD

Smoke. *see* CANNABIS

Snapper. *see* AMYL NITRITE

Snow. *see* COCAINE

Snowball. *see* MDA

Softballs. *see* Barbiturates *e.g.* AMYLOBARBITONE

Special K. *see* KETAMINE

Speed. *see* AMPHETAMINE

Splash. *see* AMPHETAMINE

Spliff. *see* CANNABIS

Sputnik. *see* CANNABIS, OPIUM (mix)

Stag. *see* AMYL NITRITE

Stardust. *see* COCAINE

Sticks. *see* CANNABIS

Strawberries. *see* LSD

Strawberry fields. *see* LSD

Stud. *see* AMYL NITRITE

Stuff. *see* CANNABIS *or* HEROIN

Sugar. *see* LSD

Sulph. *see* AMPHETAMINE *or* MORPHINE

Super K. *see* KETAMINE

Sweets. *see* AMPHETAMINE

Syrup. *see* METHADONE

Tar. *see* MORPHINE *or* OPIUM

Tea. *see* CANNABIS

Tem. *see* TEMGESIC

Temazzies. *see* TEMAZEPAM

Temmies. *see* TEMAZEPAM *or* TEMGESIC

Temple balls. *see* CANNABIS

Thai sticks. *see* CANNABIS

Tibetan gold. *see* CANNABIS

Tiger. *see* HEROIN

TNT. *see* AMYL NITRITE

Trips. *see* LSD

Truck drivers. *see* AMPHETAMINE

Uppers. *see* AMPHETAMINE

Vitamin K. *see* KETAMINE

Wacky baccy. *see* CANNABIS

Wake ups. *see* AMPHETAMINE

Wash rock. *see* COCAINE

Weed. *see* CANNABIS

White burger sauce. *see* MDA *or* MDEA *or* MDMA

White cap. *see* MDA

White cloud. *see* COCAINE

White dynamite. *see* HEROIN

White girl. *see* COCAINE

White lady. *see* COCAINE

White stuff. *see* MORPHINE *or* COCAINE

Whites. *see* AMPHETAMINE *or* MDMA

Whizz. *see* AMPHETAMINE

Whizz bomb. *see* AMPHETAMINE, LSD (mix) *or* MDMA

Window (panes). *see* LSD

Wood peckers. *see* AMPHETAMINE

XTC. *see* MDMA

Yellow submarines. *see* TEMAZEPAM

Yellows. *see* Barbiturates *e.g.* AMYLOBARBITONE

Zoom. *see* AMPHETAMINE, COCAINE, HEROIN (mix)